CHALLENGING CASES IN
Echocardiography

CHALLENGING CASES IN
Echocardiography

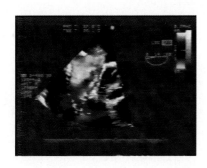
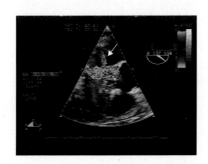
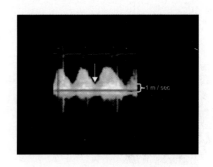

Itzhak Kronzon, MD
Professor of Medicine
Director, Non-Invasive Cardiology Laboratory
New York University School of Medicine
New York, New York

Paul A. Tunick, MD
Professor of Medicine
New York University School of Medicine
New York, New York

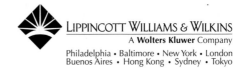
LIPPINCOTT WILLIAMS & WILKINS
A **Wolters Kluwer** Company
Philadelphia • Baltimore • New York • London
Buenos Aires • Hong Kong • Sydney • Tokyo

Acquisitions Editor: Frances Destefano
Developmental Editor: Keith Donnellan, Dovetail Content Solutions
Project Manager: Alicia Jackson
Senior Manufacturing Manager: Benjamin Rivera
Marketing Manager: Kathy Neely
Creative Director: Doug Smock
Cover Designer: Karen Kappe
Production Service: Seven Worldwide, Inc.
Printer: Quebecor World, Kingsport

© 2005 by LIPPINCOTT WILLIAMS & WILKINS
530 Walnut Street
Philadelphia, PA 19106 USA
LWW.com

Library of Congress Cataloging-in-Publication Data

Kronzon, Itzhak.
   Challenging cases in echocardiography / Itzhak Kronzon, Paul A. Tunick.
      p. ; cm.
   Includes index.
   ISBN 0-7817-5069-5 (alk. paper)
   1. Echocardiography—Case studies.   I. Tunick, Paul A.   II. Title.
[DNLM: 1. Echocardiography—Case Reports.   2. Echocardiography—Problems and
Exercises.]
RC683.5.U5K76 2005
616.1'207543—dc22   2004030549

Care has been taken to confirm the accuracy of the information presented and to describe generally accepted practices. However, the authors, editors, and publisher are not responsible for errors or omissions or for any consequences from application of the information in this book and make no warranty, expressed or implied, with respect to the currency, completeness, or accuracy of the contents of the publication. Application of the information in particular situation remains the professional responsibility of the practitioner.

The authors, editors, and publisher have exerted every effort to ensure that drug selection and dosage set forth in this text are in accordance with current recommendations and practice at the time of publication. However, in view of ongoing research, changes in government regulations, and the constant flow of information relating to drug therapy and drug reactions, the reader is urged to check the package insert for each drug for any change in indications and dosage and for added warnings and precautions. This is particularly important when the recommended agent is a new or infrequently employed drug.

Some drugs and medical devices presented in the publication have Food and Drug Administration (FDA) clearance for limited use in restricted research settings. It is the responsibility of the health care provider to ascertain the FDA status of each drug or device planned for use in their clinical practice.

10 9 8 7 6 5 4 3 2 1

Contents

Contents

Contributors

Robert M. Applebaum, MD
Assistant Professor of Medicine
New York University School of Medicine
New York, New York

Robin S. Freedberg, MD
Associate Professor of Medicine
New York University School of Medicine
New York, New York

Edward S. Katz, MD
Assistant Professor of Medicine
New York University School of Medicine
New York, New York

Ambika Nayar, MD
Assistant Professor of Medicine
New York University School of Medicine
New York, New York

Harmony R. Reynolds, MD
Assistant Professor of Medicine
New York University School of Medicine
New York, New York

Barry P. Rosenzweig, MD
Associate Professor of Medicine
New York University School of Medicine
New York, New York

Alan Shah, MD
Clinical Instructor in Medicine
New York University School of Medicine
New York, New York

Daniel M. Spevack, MD
Assistant Professor of Medicine
Albert Einstein College of Medicine
Bronx, New York

Foreword

*I*t gives me immense pleasure to introduce this book written by Drs. Itzhak Kronzon and Paul A. Tunick. This is a very unusual book. It brings to light some of the most challenging cases that one encounters when performing the practice of echocardiography.

Dr. Kronzon and Dr. Tunick are renowned cardiologists and echocardiologists. Their depth and knowledge in the field of echocardiography is immense. The readers will find the collection of cases inspiring and of significant learning. It is not every day that one encounters cases that are shown in this particular book. However, when one sees the case once he does not forget it.

The need for a book of unusual cases from the echocardiographic laboratory has now been fulfilled.

It is with great pleasure that I introduce this book to the readers and wish "happy learning."

Bijoy K. Khandheria, MD, FACC
Professor of Medicine
Mayo Clinic College of Medicine
Consultant, Cardiovascular Diseases and Internal Medicine
Mayo Clinic

Preface

_T_he history of echocardiography is filled with case reports, starting with the first demonstration by Edler and Hertz of the mitral valve in a patient with mitral stenosis, the first visualization of a myxoma by Effert, et al., and hundreds (if not thousands) of case reports in the medical literature. We have noticed that case presentations by experts in echocardiography at national and international meetings always draw a large and responsive audience. These presentations are often done with accompanying questions for the audience, sometimes with an audience-response system, which allows those attending to gauge the sentiments of the group as a whole.

This book contains a series of interesting and challenging cases that have been presented as part of the Friday morning conferences that have been held continuously over more than 10 years in the Echocardiography Laboratory at NYU. We did not intend to write a systematic textbook of echocardiography. This has been done very well several times in the past. Our book is by no means comprehensive, and many important topics and techniques are not represented. Instead, we have focused on the unusual, bizarre, difficult-to-figure-out, and instructive cases. They are intended for those who have already accumulated considerable experience using different echo modalities and for those interpreting complex diseases and unusual hemodynamic abnormalities. Echocardiography is no longer the exclusive domain of cardiologists, and this book is directed at all who utilize echocardiography in their daily practice or academic endeavors—including anesthesiologists, internists, pediatricians, intensivists, and cardiologists at every stage of their training.

Although the reader will come across recurring themes, each case may stand on its own, and the book may be digested in small or large random bites (it does not have to be read from cover to cover). Each case presentation is short and is followed by questions. The questions must be answered in the order in which they are presented, as the answers and explanations often lead to subsequent questions. The questions can be answered by referring to the single-frame images accompanying the text. The video files on the enclosed CD-ROM, which accompany many of the cases, may serve to augment the reader's appreciation of the cases involved. The video icon ☉, which appears with the case title, indicates there is at least one video clip available on the CD-ROM associated with the case. The organization of this book makes it unique, and we trust that you will find it rewarding to read.

If you are able to solve all these cases, you are doing much better than the editors! If you were stumped by some of them, we know how you feel because we were also. We hope that working through these cases will be as enjoyable as was writing them.

Itzhak Kronzon MD
Paul A. Tunick, MD

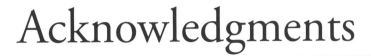

Acknowledgments

*T*he authors wish to acknowledge the superb technical, administrative, and secretarial skills of those who have worked closely with us over the years and who are largely responsible for the quality of this book. Without their devoted assistance, this project would never have been completed. Specifically, we are very grateful to Anthony Gargiulo, Mathew Varkey, Catherine Guyton, Aniko Hersko, William Sadler, Winnie Dossie, Maura Mullane, Mohamed Gasser, Anna Hamza, Maria DeGennaro, Joan O'Connell, Ayana Domingo, Shelley Nunez, Rose Maldonado, Bibi Ishmael, and our administrator and nurse, Eva Simpson. However, any errors that you may find in these cases are ours alone.

Itzhak Kronzon
Paul A. Tunick
New York, NY

CHALLENGING CASES IN

Echocardiography

1 Intra-aortic Mass After Aortic Dissection Repair

A 48-year-old man had a history of hypertension. One week ago, he was admitted to the hospital with severe chest pain. A workup at that time was diagnostic of Type A aortic dissection (involving the ascending aorta). There was no aortic insufficiency. The patient was referred for surgery, and an intimal tear was found 2 cm distal to the right coronary artery. A supra-coronary graft was placed in the ascending aorta with its distal anastomosis proximal to the innominate artery. The patient was weaned from cardiopulmonary bypass and had an uneventful immediate postoperative period. On the seventh hospital day, the patient had transient aphasia, with right-arm numbness. A transesophageal echocardiogram (TEE) was performed. There were no significant cardiac findings. The images of the descending aorta are shown below (Figures Q1.1A and Q1.1B).

QUESTION 1.1. Based on this TEE, your diagnosis is:

1. Intra-aortic thrombus
2. Artifact
3. Aortic atheroma
4. Something else

QUESTION 1.2. What would you do next?

1. Four weeks of anticoagulation, then repeat TEE
2. Reoperation
3. Consult your attorney
4. Magnetic resonance imaging

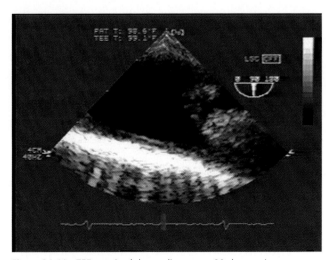

Figure Q1.1A: TEE: proximal descending aorta, 90-degree view.

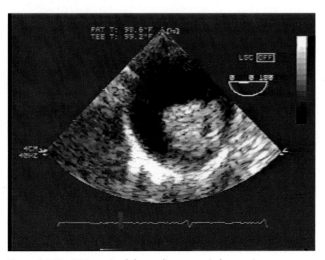

Figure Q1.1B: TEE: proximal descending aorta, 0-degree view.

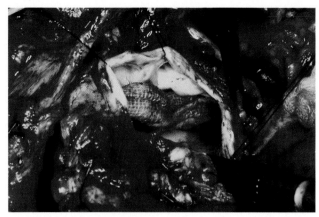

Figure A1.2A: Open proximal descending aorta (white). Note the red surgical packing filling the aorta.

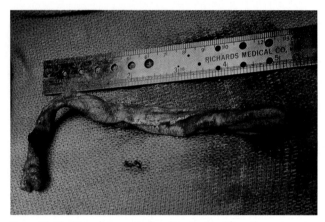

Figure A1.2B: 20-cm-long surgical packing removed from the aorta.

ANSWER 1.1. This is unlikely to be a thrombus, because of the unusual squared-off shape seen on the short-axis (0-degree) view. Furthermore, there is no evidence of aortic plaque, which would predispose to thrombosis. The appearance of the mass with a different shape on two views makes an echo-artifact unlikely. The correct answer, therefore, is 4, something else.

ANSWER 1.2. This patient has a very large mass in the aorta. Therefore, surgical removal is indicated. The correct answer is 2, reoperation. Answer 3, consulting your attorney, is always a good option, but is not specific to this case.

The patient was taken to the operating room and underwent a left thoracotomy and hypothermic circulatory arrest. The proximal descending aorta was opened, and a large, bloody mass was found. The mass appeared to be made of cloth (Figure A1.2A). Upon removal it proved to be surgical packing that measured 20 cm long (Figure A1.2B). It was attached to the distal suture line near the innominate artery and extended to the descending aorta. There were no atheromas or thrombi in the aorta.

The surgical packing was used to prevent bleeding and embolization during the case. Obviously, the sponge count was incorrect at the completion of the case.

C A S E 2 Change in Doppler Flow Pattern Following an Intervention

*T*he following two Doppler spectral tracings were recorded on transthoracic echocardiography in the same patient before and after a procedure (Figures Q2.1A and Q2.1B). Please analyze the tracings carefully, with special attention to timing, waveforms, and velocities to discern which intervention has been done. The peak velocity in the upper figure (before intervention) is 60 cm/second. The peak systolic velocity (S) in the lower figure after intervention is 30 cm/second. For both tracings, the transducer is in the second left intercostal space at the left sternal border.

QUESTION 2.1. Based on these two Doppler tracings, the most likely procedure performed was:

1. Pulmonic balloon valvuloplasty
2. Repair of aortic coarctation
3. Coronary bypass surgery
4. Tricuspid balloon valvuloplasty
5. Right inguinal herniorrhaphy

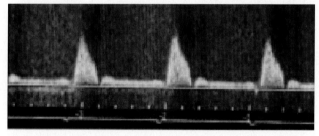

Figure Q2.1A: Transthoracic echo, preintervention, pulsed Doppler.

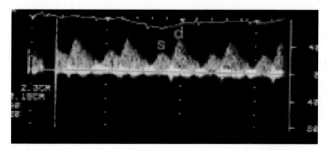

Figure Q2.1B: Transthoracic echo, postintervention, pulsed Doppler.

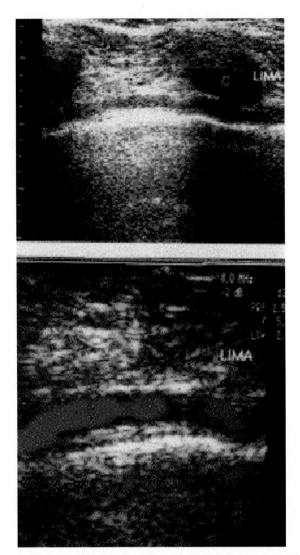

Figure A2.1: Transthoracic echocardiography with color Doppler in the lower panel.

ANSWER 2.1. Correct answer: 3, coronary artery bypass. The preprocedure (upper) tracing cannot represent pulmonic stenosis or coarctation because the systolic velocity is low (60 cm/second), and therefore the procedure was not pulmonic balloon valvuloplasty or coarctation repair. The upper tracing cannot represent tricuspid stenosis because the peak velocity is in systole, just after the QRS. If you selected herniorrhaphy, please contact the dean of your medical school and ask for your money back!

The upper tracing shows normal flow in the left internal mammary artery (LIMA) before it is anastomosed to the left anterior descending coronary artery (LAD). Note that there is predominantly systolic flow, with very low velocity diastolic flow, as seen in normal high-resistance arteries. The bottom tracing shows biphasic flow in the LIMA after it has been anastomosed to the LAD, and represents a normal biphasic pattern for LAD flow with systolic and somewhat higher diastolic peaks. This flow pattern in the LIMA indicates a patent anastomosis.

The demonstration of the LIMA and its blood flow can be obtained in 95% of patients using a high-frequency transducer (10–12 MHz) with the transducer placed on the chest wall as previously described, just above the artery (Figure A2.1). The artery can be visualized 2 cm to 3 cm under the skin, just behind the costal cartilage (C). This is a good noninvasive technique with which to evaluate graft patency after coronary artery bypass graft surgery.

3 Echo-free Space

A 75-year-old man with a previous history of coronary artery disease and bypass surgery complained of dyspnea. Workup revealed severe mitral regurgitation, and the patient underwent mitral valve replacement with a tissue prosthesis. There were no immediate postoperative problems. On the seventh postoperative day he developed dyspnea at rest and weakness. Physical examination was unremarkable.

A transthoracic echocardiogram was obtained (Figure Q3.1).

QUESTION 3.1. Based on these findings, you should order:

1. Follow-up echo in one week; drain if effusion increases or if more symptoms appear
2. Urgent needle pericardiocentesis (apical approach)
3. Urgent needle pericardiocentesis (parasternal approach)
4. Contrast echo
5. Anticoagulation with heparin, followed by warfarin (international normalized ratio = 2 to 3)

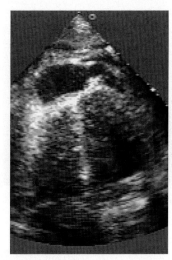

Figure Q3.1: Apical four-chamber view.

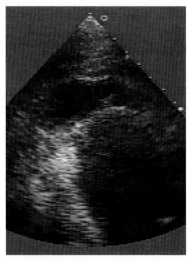

Figure A3.1A: Transthoracic echo, with contrast, apical four-chamber view.

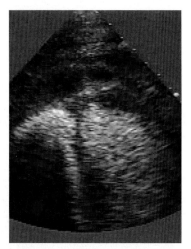

Figure A3.1B: Transthoracic echo, with contrast, apical four-chamber view, a few seconds after Figure A3.1A.

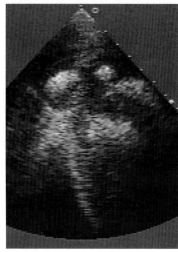

Figure A3.1C: Transthoracic echo, with contrast, apical four-chamber view, a few seconds after Figure A3.1B.

ANSWER 3.1. The correct answer is 4, contrast echo.

If you selected choices 1, 2, 3, or 5 both your patient and you are in big trouble because the echo-free space between the left ventricle (LV) apex and the chest wall is a pseudoaneurysm of the LV. Figures A3.1A, A3.1B, and A3.1C show echo-contrast, which was injected intravenously, appearing successively in the right ventricle (RV), the LV, and finally through the perforation in the LV wall into the pseudoaneurysm.

While contrast echo is an elegant way in which to make the diagnosis of LV pseudoaneurysm, it has cost us $110. The same diagnosis can be made by turning on the color or spectral turning on color or spectral Doppler (Figures A3.1D and A3.1E).

TAKE-HOME LESSON:
Never treat an echo-free space with drainage or anticoagulation without first ruling out a communication of the space with the heart.

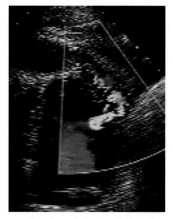

Figure A3.1D: Color Doppler shows systolic flow from the LV, through the perforation, and into the pseudoaneurysm.

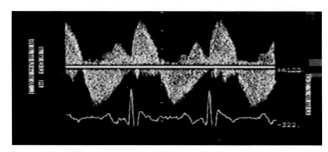

Figure A3.1E: Biphasic to-and-fro systolic and diastolic flow, into and out of the pseudoaneurysm, on continuous wave Doppler.

4 Myocardial Infarction With a New Murmur

A 74-year-old woman had an inferior wall myocardial infarction. A new murmur was heard, and a transthoracic echocardiogram was performed. The blood pressure (BP) is 130/70 mm Hg, and the lungs are clear.

QUESTION 4.1. After reviewing Figure Q4.1, what is your diagnosis?

1. Mitral regurgitation (MR), due to posteromedial papillary muscle rupture
2. Tricuspid regurgitation, due to papillary muscle rupture, with mild pulmonary hypertension
3. Ventricular septal defect (VSD)
4. Aortic stenosis

QUESTION 4.2. Now that you know the correct diagnosis, there is one more question:

What is the pulmonary artery (PA) systolic pressure?

1. Cannot be determined
2. 30 mm Hg
3. 90 mm Hg
4. 120 mm Hg

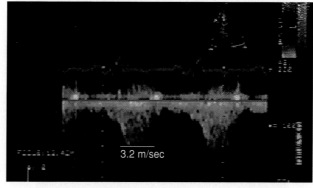

3.2 m/sec

Figure Q4.1: Spectral tracing from the continuous wave Doppler, with the transducer at the apex.

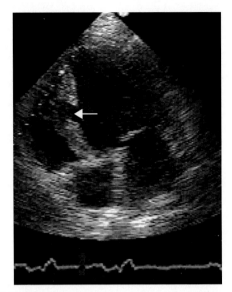

Figure A4.1A: Apical four-chamber view showing the VSD (arrow).

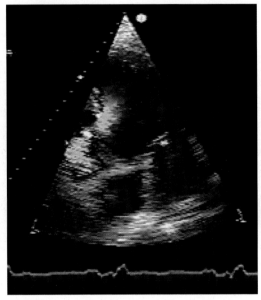

Figure A4.1B: Apical four-chamber view with color Doppler. The flow through the muscular VSD is clearly visualized.

ANSWER 4.1. The correct answer is 3, ventricular septal defect (see Figures A4.1A and A4.1B).

Number 1 is incorrect. With a systolic blood pressure of 130 mm Hg, you would expect that the velocity of mitral insufficiency would be much higher. The LV–LA pressure would be 130 minus the LA pressure. The lungs are clear; therefore the patient is not in pulmonary edema. Even with a high LA pressure of 30, the velocity of MR would be 5 m/second (a 100-mm Hg LV–LA gradient).

Number 2 is incorrect because the continuous wave (CW) Doppler shows that the flow continues from systole into diastole. The diastolic flow is low velocity, but the velocity increases during atrial contraction. Although diastolic tricuspid regurgitation is sometimes seen in patients with a slow heart rate, atrioventricular (AV) block, or an elevated right ventricular diastolic pressure, this patient is not in AV block and the sinus rate is about 70.

Number 4, aortic stenosis, is of shorter duration and does not start at the onset of the QRS, which it does in this patient. Also, aortic stenosis will not produce a "new" murmur after myocardial infarction.

It is important to remember that the basal part of the interventricular septum, as seen on the apical four-chamber view, is supplied by the right coronary artery. This is the part of the septum that may be involved in an inferior wall myocardial infarction.

ANSWER 4.2. The correct answer is 3, 90 mm Hg. The CW shows that the jet velocity in systole is 3.2 m/sec and $4 \times v^2$ is 40. Therefore, the gradient between the LV and right ventricle (RV) is 40 mm Hg. Because the RV and PA systolic pressures are the same (assume there is no pulmonic stenosis) the gradient between the LV and PA is also 40 mm Hg. Because the BP is 130 mm Hg, and this is also the LV pressure in the absence of aortic stenosis, the PA systolic pressure is 130–40, or 90 mm Hg.

C A S E

5 What Was the Procedure?

A 17-year-old boy had a surgical procedure. Two images were taken before and after the procedure (Figures Q5.1A and Q5.1B). The sample volume of these two pulsed Doppler tracings was at the same site for both images.

QUESTION 5.1. What was the procedure?

1. Aortic valve replacement
2. Atrial septal defect (ASD) repair
3. Tricuspid annuloplasty
4. Aortic coarctation repair

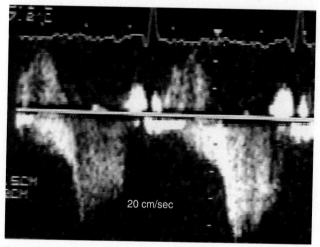

Figure Q5.1A: Preprocedure.

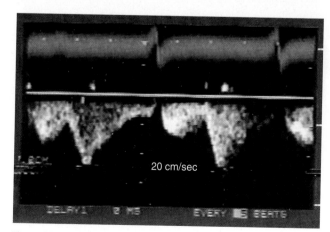

Figure Q5.1B: Postprocedure.

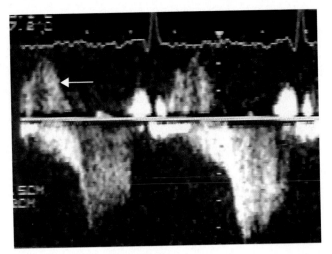

Figure A5.1A: Same as Figure Q5.1A.

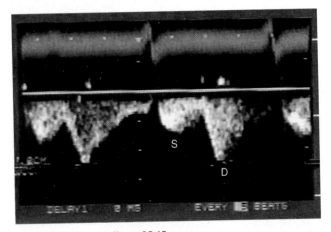

Figure A5.1B: Same as Figure Q5.1B.

ANSWER 5.1. Correct answer: 1, aortic valve replacement. These pulsed Doppler tracings were taken with the sample volume in the left anterior descending coronary artery, during intraoperative transesophageal echocardiography (TEE). The patient had severe aortic stenosis. Because of that, the systolic pressure in the left ventricle was much higher than that in the aorta. This resulted in systolic reversal of coronary blood flow (Figure A5.1A).

After aortic valve replacement, the coronary flow pattern reverted to normal, with antegrade flow in both systole (S) and diastole (D) (Figure A5.1B) (the flow velocity in diastole is normally higher in the left anterior descending coronary artery).

The procedure was not an ASD repair. Although an ASD may have bidirectional flow, there should be no flow after the ASD is repaired. After a tricuspid annuloplasty, there cannot be both systolic and diastolic flow in the same direction. In coarctation of the aorta, there is a systolic gradient across the coarctation. Here the maximal systolic velocity preop is only 40 cm/sec.

TAKE-HOME LESSON:
The symptom of angina in a patient with aortic stenosis may be, in part, related to a systolic "coronary steal," with retrograde systolic flow as is seen in this patient.

6 A 27-Year-Old Patient With a Murmur

Seven years ago this 27-year-old man had a Ross procedure for severe aortic valve disease (stenosis and insufficiency). For the past 2 years, a systolic ejection murmur was heard at the upper left sternal border, which increased in intensity with inspiration. There was no diastolic murmur. The patient was New York Heart Association (NYHA) class I. The blood pressure was 120/80 mm Hg. The following echocardiogram was obtained with the transducer at the upper left sternal border (Figures Q6.1 and Q6.2).

The proximal isovelocity surface area (PISA) radius is 1 cm; the aliasing velocity was set at 72 cm/second.

QUESTION 6.1. What is the pulmonic valve area?

1. 0.3 cm2
2. 0.6 cm2
3. 0.9 cm2
4. 1.2 cm2

QUESTION 6.2. The reason for the intermittent antegrade pulmonic flow during end-diastole (arrow in Figure Q6.2) is

1. Pulmonic regurgitation
2. The right atrium (RA) A wave exceeds pulmonary artery diastolic pressure
3. Pulmonic stenosis is not severe
4. The patient has right ventricle (RV) failure

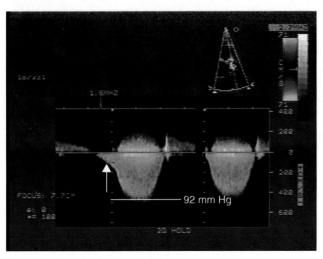

Figure Q6.1: Continuous wave Doppler.

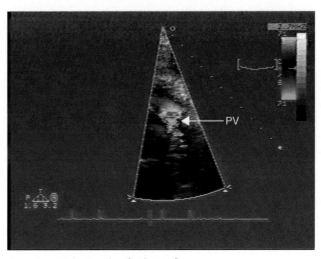

Figure Q6.2: Color Doppler of pulmonic flow.

ANSWER 6.1. Correct answer: 3, 0.9 cm². The calculation of valve area using PISA is as follows:

$$\text{Valve Area} = \frac{\text{Maximal Valve Flow Rate (MVFR)}}{\text{Maximal Valve Flow Velocity}}.$$

The Maximal Valve Flow Rate is $2\pi r^2$ (the PISA hemisphere area) multiplied by the aliasing velocity. Therefore the MVFR is $2 \times 1 \times 1 \times 3.14 \times 72 = 452$ cc/second.

The peak gradient is 92 mm Hg. Therefore the Maximal Valve Flow Velocity (from the continuous wave Doppler) is approximately 4.8 m/second, or 480 cm/second ($\Delta p = 4v^2$, simplified Bernouilli equation).

The Valve Area is 452 / 480 = 0.9 cm².

ANSWER 6.2. Correct answer: 2, RA A wave exceeds pulmonary artery diastolic pressure. With severe PS, the pulmonary artery pressure is low. With inspiration, and the subsequent increase in return to the right atrium, the atrial A wave rises above the (low) pulmonary artery diastolic pressure. This leads to diastolic (premature) opening of the pulmonic valve and antegrade flow across the valve in end-diastole.

7 Dyspnea on Exertion

A 24-year-old woman presented with progressive shortness of breath on exertion. According to her mother she had a history of a febrile illness in childhood. An echocardiogram was ordered (Figures Q7.1A and Q7.1B).

QUESTION 7.1. This study suggests:

1. Loeffler's hypereosinophilic syndrome with endocardial thickening
2. Rheumatic mitral stenosis (MS)
3. Congenital heart disease
4. Left atrial myxoma

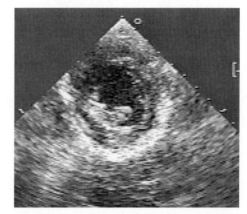

Figure Q7.1A: Short-axis parasternal view of the left ventricle.

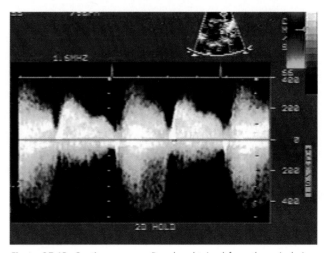

Figure Q7.1B: Continuous wave Doppler obtained from the apical view, recording transmitral flow.

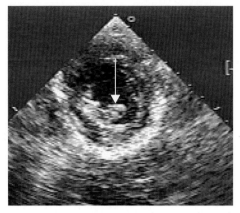

Figure A7.1A: Same view as Figure Q7.1A demonstrating single papillary muscle.

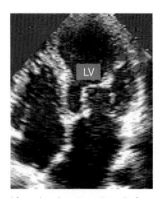

Figure A7.1B: Apical four-chamber view, diastolic frame.

ANSWER 7.1. Correct answer: 3, congenital heart disease.

The patient suffers from mitral stenosis. The continuous wave Doppler shows a large diastolic gradient across the mitral valve (the peak diastolic velocity is 2.8 m/sec and the mean gradient is 17 mm Hg). The continuous wave Doppler also shows mitral regurgitation.

Although most patients with mitral stenosis have rheumatic heart disease, this is not the case in our patient. The short-axis view clearly shows a single papillary muscle located at 6 o'clock (arrow in Figure A7.1A).

This is characteristic of a parachute mitral valve, in which all of the chordae tendinae are attached to a single papillary muscle. This creates a funnel-shaped left ventricular inflow with a gradient between the left atrium and left ventricle.

Figure A7.1B shows thin, noncalcified mitral leaflets. All of the chordae from both the anterior and posterior mitral leaflet are attached to the single papillary muscle.

TAKE-HOME LESSON:

All that glitters is not gold! (Not all mitral stenosis is rheumatic.) About 1% of MS cases are congenital, and the most common anatomy in these patients is a parachute mitral valve.

8 Progressive Dyspnea on Exertion

A 71-year-old man complained of progressive dyspnea on exertion, now occurring after walking only one-half block. His past history was positive for a myocardial infarction 11 years previously, with no angina subsequently, and colon cancer 3 years ago. Because of his history of myocardial infarction, an echocardiogram was obtained (Figure Q8.1).

QUESTION 8.1. The presumptive diagnosis is

1. Left ventricular (LV) pseudoaneurysm
2. Left ventricular aneurysm
3. Pleural effusion
4. Pericardial effusion
5. Ebstein's anomaly

QUESTION 8.2. The next step should be

1. Exercise echo
2. Dobutamine stress echo
3. Thoracentesis
4. LV angiogram
5. Another test

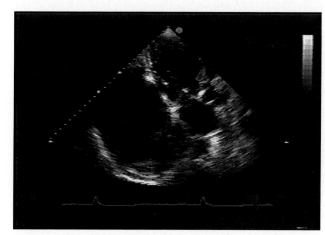

Figure Q8.1: Transthoracic echo, apical long-axis view.

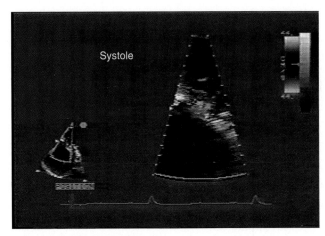

Figure A8.2A: Transthoracic echo, apical long-axis view, with color Doppler, systolic frame.

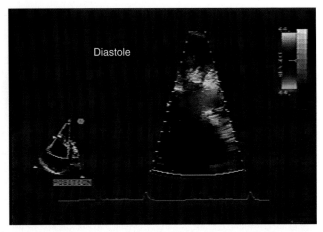

Figure A8.2B: Transthoracic echo, apical long-axis view, with color Doppler, diastolic frame.

ANSWER 8.1. Correct answer: 1, a huge (17-cm) LV pseudoaneurysm. There is a large hole in the posterior wall, leading to the large collection of blood contained by the pericardium. The space is not delimited by the LV wall (as would be the case in a true aneurysm). Although Ebstein's anomaly may be the cause of an extremely large atrialized portion of the right ventricle, the space in this case is posterior to the left ventricle, not anterior to it, and no tricuspid valve is seen in this view.

ANSWER 8.2. Correct answer: 5, another test. The other test is taken by turning on the color Doppler (Figures A8.2A and A8.2B).

Color Doppler shows that the large echo-free space adjacent to the left ventricle is actually a giant left ventricular pseudoaneurysm. Note that there is flow from the LV into the pseudoaneurysm in systole (blue) and then back into the LV in diastole (red). The hole (communication) between the ventricle and the pseudoaneurysm is large (about 4 cm). This is atypical, as is the giant size of the pseudoaneurysm.

The other answers are invasive (LV angiogram), nonspecific (exercise or dobutamine echo), or dangerous (thoracentesis).

TAKE-HOME LESSON:

Although LV pseudoaneurysms should be resected when they are discovered just after infarction, some may be chronic, and (as in this case) giant! An echo-free space around the heart should always be explored with color Doppler.

9 Different Left Ventricular Gradients

A 27-year-old patient has had a murmur since birth. He is now being evaluated for a syncopal episode after a hot shower.

A continuous wave (CW) Doppler was obtained with the transducer at the apex (Figure Q9.1). The vertical distance between 2 dots is 1 m/sec.

QUESTION 9.1. What is the diagnosis?

1. Mitral regurgitation
2. Fixed left ventricular outflow tract (LVOT) obstruction
3. Dynamic LVOT obstruction
4. Combined dynamic and fixed outflow obstruction
5. All of the above

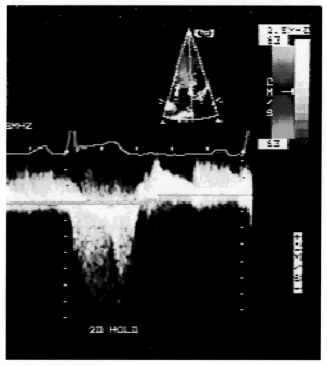

Figure Q9.1: CW Doppler.

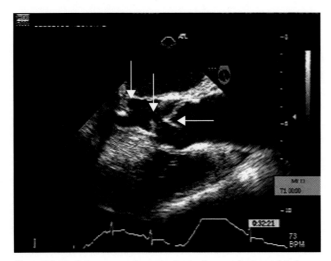

Figure A9.1A: 2-D transesophageal echocardiogram, horizontal 0-degree plane.

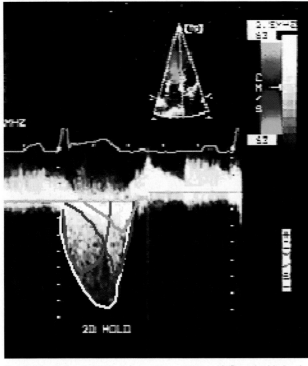

Figure A9.1B: Same CW Doppler as Figure Q9.1, with flows highlighted.

ANSWER 9.1. Correct answer: 5, all of the above. See Figures A9.1A and A9.1B.

Figure A9.1A shows that there is

1. Systolic anterior motion of the mitral valve, creating left ventricular outflow obstruction (left vertical arrow)

2. A subvalvular membrane (right vertical arrow) several millimeters below the aortic valve (horizontal arrow)

If you look closely again at the continuous wave Doppler (Figure A9.1B), you can distinguish four different flows within the systolic signal.

The blue-outlined signal, peaking in late systole, represents a dynamic LVOT gradient caused by mitral systolic anterior motion. This is a late-systolic velocity of approximately 4 m/second. The red-outlined signal, peaking in midsystole, is characteristic of fixed LVOT obstruction caused by the subvalvular membrane. The white-outlined signal is of longer duration than the previous two and reaches a velocity of 6.3 m/second. This is mitral insufficiency. There is also a green-outlined signal (difficult to see), which apparently represents the flow velocity proximal to the first obstruction (the first obstruction is due to mitral systolic anterior motion). This was similar in shape and velocity to a pulsed Doppler recording at this site.

Continuous wave Doppler has no depth resolution (no range-gating, or sample volume, as does pulsed Doppler); therefore, all of the velocities in the path of the beam are superimposed on one another. As a result, the two subvalvular stenoses (due to mitral systolic anterior motion and to the fixed subaortic membrane) have velocities that appear within the fastest and widest envelope (mitral regurgitation).

TAKE-HOME LESSON:

Your CW Doppler frequently contains more than one velocity signal, with two or more signals superimposed on each other. Always consider performing CW Doppler with a lower gain setting, to avoid hiding the superimposed velocities.

10 Concerned Mother

*T*he mother of a 14-year-old boy is concerned about the risk of sudden death among young athletes, which she has read about in the newspapers. The child is asymptomatic, even with strenuous exercise. An echocardiogram is performed (Figures Q10.1A and Q10.1B).

QUESTION 10.1. Assuming that the rest of the study is normal, should the child be allowed to continue strenuous exercise?

1. Yes, the echo findings shown are normal
2. Yes, he has an atrial septal defect (ASD)
3. No, he has a risk of oxygen desaturation with exercise
4. No, he has a risk of sudden death with exercise

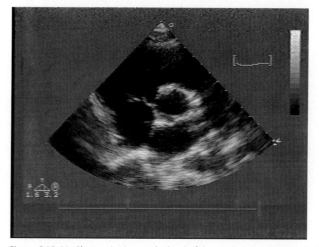

Figure Q10.1A: Short-axis view at the level of the aortic valve-sinuses of Valsalva.

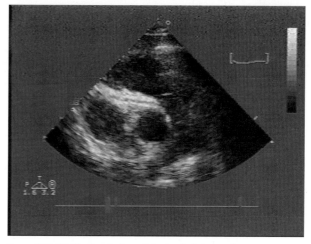

Figure Q10.1B: Short-axis view at the level of the aortic root.

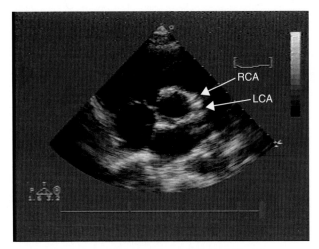

Figure A10.1A: Same image as Figure Q10.1A. RCA, right coronary artery; LCA, left coronary artery.

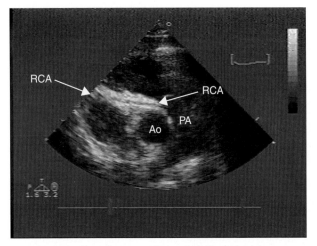

Figure A10.1B: Same image as Figure Q10.1B. RCA, right coronary artery; LCA, left coronary artery; Ao, aorta; PA, pulmonary artery.

ANSWER 10.1. Correct answer: 4, no, he has a risk of sudden death with exercise (Figures A10.1A and A10.1B).

This patient has anomalous origin of the right coronary artery (RCA) from the left sinus of Valsalva. Figure A10.1A shows a short-axis view of the aorta at the level of the sinuses of Valsalva. Note the two ostia—one for the normal left coronary artery and the other for the anomalous right coronary artery.

This anomalous RCA takes a course between the aorta and the pulmonary artery before proceeding to the right (arrows, Figure A10.1B). With vigorous exercise, both great vessels become larger and the anomalous artery may be compressed, which may cause myocardial ischemia and sudden death.

Anomalous origin of the left coronary artery also occurs. The majority of patients with anomalous coronary arteries who die suddenly were previously asymptomatic. Anomalous coronary arteries occur in up to 0.2% of child athletes. Treatment options include avoidance of exercise, coronary artery bypass grafting, and possible reimplantation. The management of asymptomatic patients with anomalous coronary arteries (such as this patient) is controversial. Hypertrophic obstructive cardiomyopathy is another echocardiographic constellation of findings to look for in young athletes that may also put them at risk for sudden death on exertion.

CASE *11* Can You Interpret This Doppler Spectral Tracing?

*A*n elderly patient is having an echocardiogram because of palpitation. He is otherwise asymptomatic. A surprising Doppler spectral tracing is obtained with the transducer at the apex (Figure Q11.1):

QUESTION 11.1. The correct diagnosis is

1. Pulmonic stenosis and regurgitation
2. Aortic regurgitation (AR)
3. Mitral stenosis
4. Ventricular septal defect (VSD)

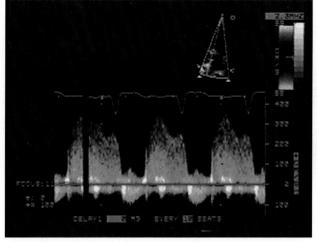

Figure Q11.1: Transthoracic echo, apical window, continuous wave Doppler.

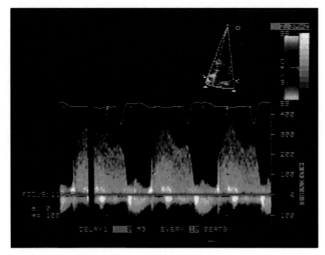

Figure A11.1A: Same as Figure Q11.1.

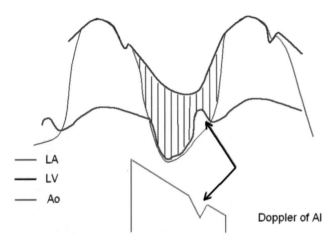

—— LA
—— LV
—— Ao

Doppler of AI

Figure A11.1B: Hemodynamic drawing of intracardiac pressures (top) and Doppler tracing of aortic insufficiency (AI) (bottom).

ANSWER 11.1. Correct answer: 2, aortic regurgitation.

At first glance, the shape of this spectral Doppler may suggest mitral stenosis in a patient with NSR. However, if this is mitral stenosis, and the gradient reaches 50 mm Hg, the patient must be symptomatic (dyspneic). Also note that the diastolic flow starts immediately after, and ends immediately before, the systolic flow. If this were mitral stenosis, one would expect a delay between aortic closure and mitral opening (isovolumetric relaxation) and a delay between mitral closure and aortic opening. This is not the case, and therefore the diastolic flow velocity displayed is that of aortic regurgitation, and not mitral stenosis.

The spectral tracing of pulmonic regurgitation usually cannot be obtained from the apical window. In addition, there is no systolic high velocity (no pulmonic stenosis), therefore this is not the right answer. VSD is never associated with a high-velocity diastolic flow; the diastolic flow between the left ventricle (LV) and right ventricle (RV) in a VSD is low velocity.

The unusual feature is the striking "A dip" noted in the AR spectral tracing in end-diastole (arrow, Figure A11.1A). This occurs because the patient must have marked elevation of left ventricular pressure during atrial contraction. The increase in left ventricular pressure at end-diastole decreases the end-diastolic gradient between the aorta and the LV (Figure A11.1B). Such an A dip may often be seen in the spectral tracing of pulmonic regurgitation, but is quite unusual with aortic regurgitation (ordinarily, aortic pressure is much higher than pulmonary artery pressure and the relative increase in ventricular pressure during atrial contraction is smaller).

12 Weight Loss

A 79-year-old man presented with a 15-pound weight loss over 2 months. Physical examination revealed hepatomegaly, ascites, and ankle edema.

A Doppler tracing was obtained from the subxiphoid view (Figure Q12.1).

QUESTION 12.1. The spectral Doppler shows a blood flow characteristic of:

1. Atrial septal defect (ASD) with left-to-right shunt
2. 70% stenosis of the right coronary artery
3. Venous obstruction
4. Arterio-venous fistula
5. Left ventricular (LV) pseudoaneurysm

QUESTION 12.2. In addition, the apical four-chamber view appears in Figure Q12.2.

Based on Figures Q12.1 and Q12.2, your diagnosis is

1. Hepatoma
2. Right atrial myxoma
3. Right atrial fibroelastoma
4. Atrial septal defect
5. Carcinoid heart disease

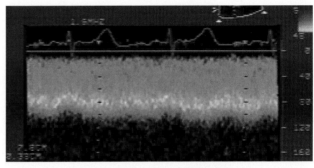

Figure Q12.1: Doppler tracing from the subxiphoid view.

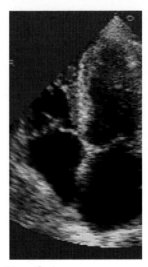

Figure Q12.2: Apical four-chamber view.

ANSWER 12.1. Correct answer: 3, venous obstruction. This spectral tracing (Figure Q12.1) does not represent that of an atrial septal defect. Although there is flow throughout systole and diastole, the flow through an ASD always decreases after the QRS and this flow velocity remains constant. The flow from a left-to-right shunt would also be toward the transducer from the subxiphoid view, and the flow in this case is below the baseline (away from the transducer).

Although coronary flow may occasionally be seen from the subxiphoid view, it always has two waves (systolic and diastolic). Right coronary flow has a more prominent systolic wave than does left coronary flow. The flow in this case is continuous and does not have phasic variation.

An arterio-venous fistula flow is also continuous; however the velocities are higher, representing the gradient between a systemic artery and vein. In addition, the systolic velocity will be higher than the diastolic velocity, as systemic arterial pressure is significantly higher in systole than in diastole.

Flow seen in a left ventricular pseudoaneurysm is biphasic and in opposite directions in systole and diastole (into the pseudoaneurysm in systole, and back into the LV in diastole).

Also, none of the above diagnoses (except 3) have anything to do with the patient's clinical presentation (weight loss).

Figure Q12.1 is characteristic of venous obstruction. There is continuous flow throughout the cardiac cycle, at a velocity of approximately 1.1 m/second. The characteristic antegrade systolic and diastolic waves of normal venous flow, as well as the retrograde A wave during atrial contraction, are absent. The overall velocity is higher than normal. Normally the systolic wave in a systemic vein is up to 80 cm/second and the diastolic wave is up to 60 cm/second.

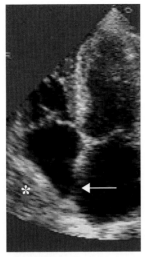

Figure A12.2A: Same view as Figure Q12.2.

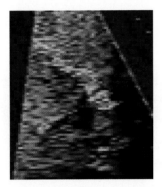

Figure A12.2B: Aliased color flow within the hepatic veins.

ANSWER 12.2. The correct answer relating to the four-chamber view is 1, hepatoma.

A right atrial tumor, such as a myxoma or a papillary fibroelastoma, is intracavitary. A myxoma is usually attached to the atrial septum, and a fibroelastoma may be on a valve or on a cardiac wall. The four-chamber view in this case shows external compression of the right atrium (asterisk, Figure A12.2A).

There is the commonly seen "dropout" (arrow, Figure A12.2A) in the atrial septum on this four-chamber view, which does not necessarily represent pathology. In addition, the right atrium is not enlarged, as it would be in a patient with an ASD, ascites, edema, or hepatomegaly.

The tricuspid valve appears normal and not thickened as it would be in carcinoid involvement. Also, in patients with carcinoid tumors affecting the right heart, right atrial enlargement would be present in a patient with edema, ascites, etc.

Therefore the most likely diagnosis is hepatoma with external compression of the right atrium and intrahepatic veins.

Figure A12.2B shows high-velocity aliased, turbulent color flow within the hepatic veins, which are externally compressed by the hepatoma. This was confirmed by liver biopsy.

The patient's presentation with ascites and edema is characteristic of inferior vena cava syndrome, which has been confirmed by Doppler echocardiography.

CASE 13 A Patient With an Asymptomatic Murmur

*A*n M-mode image was obtained in an asymptomatic 34-year-old man referred because of a murmur (Figure Q13.1).

QUESTION13.1. Which valve is imaged on this transthoracic, M-mode echocardiogram?

1. Mitral valve
2. Tricuspid valve
3. Aortic valve
4. Pulmonic valve

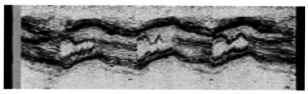

Figure Q13.1: M-mode echo.

QUESTION 13.2. Now that you know what valve it is, what is the diagnosis?

1. Ventricular bigeminy
2. Left bundle branch block
3. Hypertrophic obstructive cardiomyopathy
4. Hemochromatosis

QUESTION 13.3. The left ventricular outflow tract (LVOT) gradient in this patient is likely to be

1. 0 mm Hg
2. 20 mm Hg
3. 50 mm Hg
4. ≥ 100 mm Hg

QUESTION 13.4. What is the other likely abnormality present in this patient?

1. Mitral regurgitation (MR)
2. Aortic stenosis (AS)
3. Right ventricular outflow obstruction
4. Coarctation of the aorta

QUESTION 13.5. Last food for thought: In a patient with arterial blood pressure of 120/80 mm Hg, who has the combination of hypertrophic obstructive cardiomyopathy, aortic stenosis, and mitral regurgitation, which flow will have the fastest velocity?

1. Aortic stenosis
2. Mitral regurgitation
3. LVOT obstruction
4. It's not possible to say

ANSWER 13.1. The correct answer is 3, aortic valve.

At first glance, one might suspect that the valve imaged is an atrioventricular (AV) valve since AV valves open early in diastole, close partially in mid-diastole, and then open again in late diastole. There are two clues that should make it apparent that this is not the mitral or tricuspid valve. First, the valve opens in systole, not diastole. Secondly, the walls surrounding the valve are thin (like a vessel) rather than thick (like a ventricle). The valve is seen opening perpendicular to the plane of the echo beam. This approach normally is not possible for the pulmonic valve from transthoracic windows.

ANSWER 13.2. The correct answer is 3, hypertrophic obstructive cardiomyopathy. This M-mode echocardiogram is suggestive of dynamic subaortic stenosis. At the beginning of systole, aortic valve opening is normal. As systole progresses, there is obstruction to outflow (due to mitral systolic anterior motion, Figure A13.2) and the aortic valve begins to close in mid-systole (arrow, Figure A13.2). As systole progresses, left ventricular (LV) pressure rises enough to overcome the obstruction and the aortic valve opens fully again. Left bundle branch block alters the sequence of contraction but does not cause midsystolic aortic valve closure. Ventricular bigeminy is not seen on the ECG. The sepia color of the M-mode echo should not be confused with hemochromatosis.

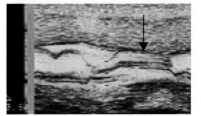

Figure A13.2: M-mode echo showing severe septal hypertrophy and mitral systolic anterior motion.

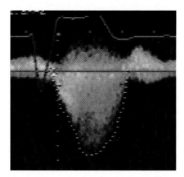

Figure A13.3: Continuous wave Doppler of the LVOT gradient (approximately 120 mm Hg).

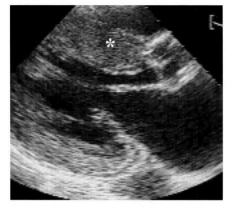

Figure A13.4A: Parasternal long axis, showing severe asymmetrical septal hypertrophy (*).

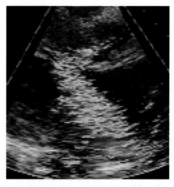

Figure A13.4B: Same view as Figure A13.4A, with color Doppler showing perpendicular jets of LVOT flow and MR.

ANSWER 13.3. The correct answer is 4, ≥ 100 mm Hg. The mitral systolic anterior motion reaches the septum and stays in contact with it throughout systole. This causes severe LVOT obstruction with a large gradient (Figure A13.3). When the mitral valve does not reach the septum, the gradient is absent or small. When the mitral valve reaches the septum but stays in contact with it only briefly (< 40% of systole), the gradient is usually not severe.

ANSWER 13.4. Correct answer: 1, mitral regurgitation. The mitral systolic anterior motion present in patients with hypertrophic obstructive cardiomyopathy frequently distorts the mitral valve and interferes with its coaptation. This (along with the increased LV pressure in systole due to LVOT obstruction) leads to significant mitral regurgitation. The MR jet is typically perpendicular to the outflow jet, and both appear as aliased, high-velocity turbulent jets on color Doppler (Figures A13.4A and A13.4B).

Aortic stenosis can occur in combination with hypertrophic obstructive cardiomyopathy, however this is incidental (they don't share a common etiology) and the likelihood that they will occur in the same patient is low. Right ventricular outflow obstruction may be associated with hypertrophic obstructive cardiomyopathy, but it is rare (< 5%). Coarctation may be associated with bicuspid aortic valve and subaortic membrane, but not with hypertrophic obstructive cardiomyopathy.

ANSWER 13.5. Correct answer: 2, mitral regurgitation. The velocity of a particular flow depends on the driving gradient of pressure. Let's call the LVOT gradient "A" and the aortic valve gradient "B." When a patient has the combination mentioned (hypertrophic obstructive cardiomyopathy, aortic stenosis, and mitral regurgitation), and a blood pressure of 120 systolic, the pressure gradient between the LV and the left atrium (LA) (the gradient of MR) will be 120 plus "A" plus "B", minus the LA pressure. Because the left atrial pressure is always smaller than 120, the MR jet will have the fastest velocity. For example, if the blood pressure is 120, the LVOT gradient is 60, and the aortic gradient is 80, then the left ventricular pressure is 260. If the left atrial pressure is 10, then the MR gradient will be 250. With these gradients, the velocities will be: LVOT = approximately 3.8 m/second, AS = 4.5 m/second, and MR = 7.9 m/second.

14 Massive Cardiomegaly in an Asymptomatic Patient

A 27-year-old man is referred because of a markedly enlarged cardiac silhouette on x-ray. He has known of an abnormal electrocardiogram (EKG) for many years.

An echocardiogram is obtained (Figures A14.1A-C).

QUESTION 14.1. The diagnosis is

1. Secundum atrial septal defect (ASD)
2. Sinus venosus ASD
3. Ebstein's anomaly
4. Cor triatriatum dexter

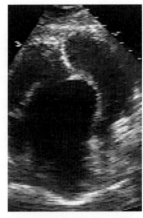

Figure Q14.1A: Apical four-chamber view.

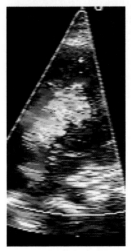

Figure Q14.1B: Same apical view as Figure Q14.1A, with color Doppler.

QUESTION 14.2. The EKG of this patient most likely shows:

1. Right ventricular hypertrophy
2. Left anterior hemiblock (LAHB)
3. Deep T-wave inversions in V4-6
4. Wolff-Parkinson-White syndrome (WPW)

QUESTION 14.3. Another echocardiographic finding that may be present in Ebstein's anomaly is

1. Right-to-left shunting
2. Left-to-right shunting
3. Pulmonary hypertension
4. Low left ventricle (LV) ejection fraction

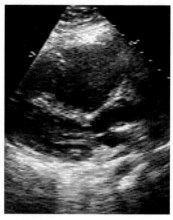

Figure Q14.1C: Long-axis view.

ANSWER 14.1. Correct answer: 3, Ebstein's anomaly. In Figure A14.1A, the tricuspid septal leaflet can be seen more than halfway toward the right ventricular (RV) apex (arrow), the cardinal abnormality in Ebstein's.

Because of this, the coaptation of the tricuspid valve is faulty, resulting in tricuspid regurgitation, which also starts deep in the right ventricle rather than at the tricuspid annulus (as seen in Figure A14.1B, white arrow). The yellow arrow in Figure A14.1B points to the mitral valve.

The displacement of the tricuspid valve results in a large chamber that has atrial hemodynamics (on the atrial side of the displaced valve). However, at least one wall is made up of right ventricular myocardium (arrows, Figure A14.1C), and will therefore have a ventricular electrogram. This chamber is referred to as the "atrialized" portion of the right ventricle (ARV).

ANSWER 14.2. The correct answer is 4, WPW (ventricular pre-excitation). This is present in approximately 30% of patients with Ebstein's anomaly.

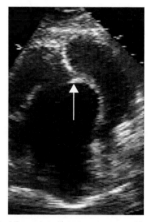

Figure A14.1A: Apical four-chamber view, same as Figure Q14.1A.

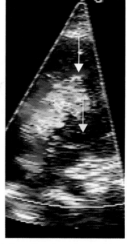

Figure A14.1B: Apical four-chamber view, with color Doppler, same as Figure Q14.1B.

ANSWER 14.3. The correct answer is 1, right-to-left shunting. Because patent foramen ovale (PFO) is a common finding in adults, and a patient with Ebstein's may more commonly have PFO, it may become stretched open, resulting in right-to-left shunting. This is aggravated by high right atrium pressure due to tricuspid regurgitation (TR). A left-to-right shunt is uncommon. Ebstein's anomaly is one of the very few congenital defects in which the patient may be cyanotic with a normal pulmonary artery (PA) pressure.

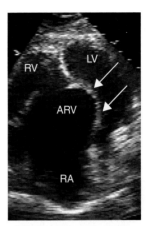

Figure A14.1C: Apical four-chamber view, same as Figure Q14.1A.

TAKE-HOME LESSON:

Always pay attention to the site at which TR starts. The tricuspid annulus is normally more apical than the mitral annulus, but this difference is normally not more than 1.5 cm. The leaflets of the tricuspid valve are not always well visualized, and if TR is noted to start toward the RV apex, this points to the diagnosis of Ebstein's anomaly.

15 Shortness of Breath

A 61-year-old man is referred for echocardiography because of dyspnea on 3 blocks' exertion. On physical examination there was a diastolic rumble at the apex. Spectral Doppler tracings were obtained from the apical view (Figures Q15.1A and Q15.1B).

QUESTION 15.1. Based on these two Doppler tracings, the diagnosis is

1. Cor triatriatum
2. Rheumatic mitral stenosis
3. Parachute mitral valve
4. Carcinoid, in a patient with congenitally corrected (L) transposition

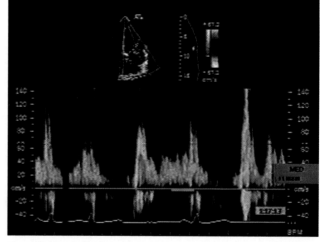

Figure Q15.1A: Pulsed Doppler with the sample volume in the left ventricle at the tips of the mitral leaflets.

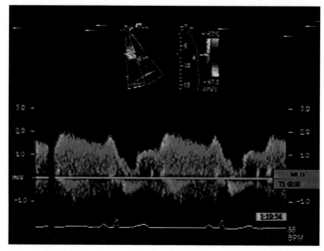

Figure Q15.1B: Continuous wave Doppler along the same plane as in Figure Q15.1A.

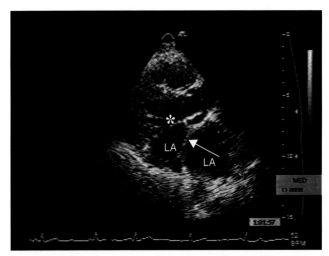

Figure A15.1A: Parasternal long-axis view. Note that there is a membrane within the left atrium (arrow). The mitral valve (*) is thin and appears to be normal.

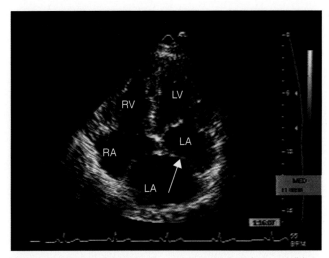

Figure A15.1B: Apical four-chamber view. Note that there are "three atria" with a membrane dividing the left atrium (arrow).

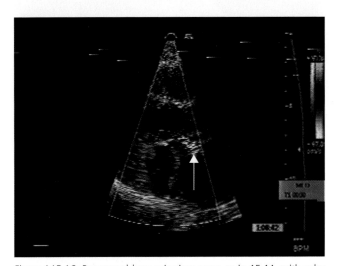

Figure A15.1C: Parasternal long-axis view, same as in 15.1A, with color Doppler added. Note that there is an aliased turbulent jet going through a hole in the membrane (arrow) toward the mitral valve. The jet loops downward under the mitral valve (blue) and back up (red).

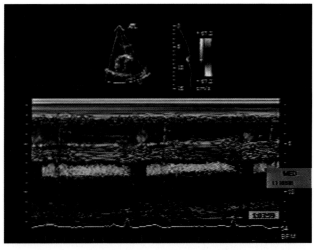

Figure A15.1D: Color M-mode of the flow through the hole in the membrane. Note that the color jet is continuous throughout systole and diastole, with a short cessation after the QRS (after atrial contraction, during atrial relaxation, as seen on the spectral tracing in Figure Q15.1B).

ANSWER 15.1. Correct answer: 1, cor triatriatum. Figure Q15.1A shows that there is no valvular mitral stenosis (making choices 2, 3, and 4 incorrect). The velocity is low, and the deceleration time (pressure half-time) is normal, ruling out valvular mitral stenosis.

Figure Q15.1B shows an abnormal gradient somewhere along the path of the ultrasound beam. The gradient is present in both diastole and systole, with a brief cessation after atrial contraction (during atrial relaxation). Therefore although there is no gradient across the mitral valve, there is a gradient within the left atrium, as seen in cor triatriatum.

See Figures A15.1A through A15.1D for further imaging and discussion.

TAKE-HOME LESSON:

On history and physical it is difficult to distinguish cor triatriatum from valvular mitral stenosis. Echocardiography can define the anatomic abnormality and can also show that the gradient within the atrium continues in systole (unlike mitral stenosis).

CASE 16 A 62-Year-Old Woman With Disseminated Intravascular Coagulation

A 62-year-old woman with a history of chronic obstructive pulmonary disease and a myocardial infarction 1 year ago, is admitted with shortness of breath. Physical examination revealed anasarca. Laboratory evaluation showed a low platelet count, an increased International Normalized Ratio, and fibrin split products consistent with disseminated intravascular coagulation (DIC). An echocardiogram was obtained (Figures Q16.1A and Q16.1B).

QUESTION 16.1. What is your diagnosis?

1. Noncompaction of the left ventricle
2. Left ventricular (LV) aneurysm
3. Left ventricular pseudoaneurysm
4. Loeffler's syndrome (hypereosinophilic syndrome)

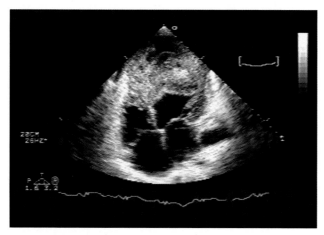

Figure Q16.1A: Apical four-chamber view, systolic frame.

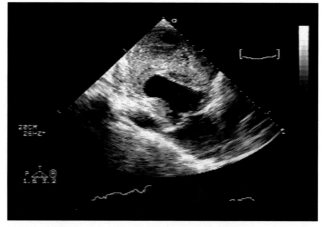

Figure Q16.1B: Two-chamber view.

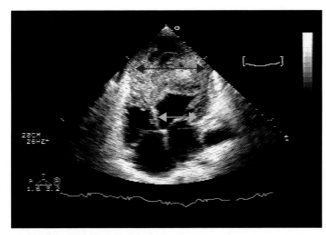

Figure A16.1: Same as Figure Q16.1A.

ANSWER 16.1. Correct answer: 2, LV aneurysm. Note that the left ventricle is ballooned out, and wider at the apex in systole (red arrow) than at the base (yellow arrow). The aneurysm is filled with clot and does not contract (see accompanying video). In Loeffler's syndrome there may be a similar filling defect, but wall motion is not absent and the apex is not dilated. This is not noncompaction because in noncompaction there is increased LV trabeculation, not marked dilatation. In pseudoaneurysm, there is a narrow neck.

This huge clot within a left ventricular aneurysm is unusual. The DIC picture actually represents consumption coagulopathy (Figure A16.1).

17 Shortness of Breath in a Patient With a Mitral Valve Prosthesis

A 67-year-old woman had a mitral St. Jude's prosthesis and a DDD pacemaker implanted 2 years ago because of severe mitral stenosis. Her symptoms improved, but she still complained of mild dyspnea on exertion. On physical examination there were crisp valve clicks and a 2/6 systolic ejection murmur audible at the left sternal border and apex.

QUESTION 17.1. The following echocardiogram was obtained (Figure Q17.1). What is your diagnosis?

1. Valvular aortic stenosis
2. Subvalvular aortic stenosis
3. Supravalvular aortic stenosis
4. Low cardiac output

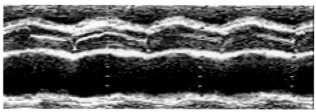

Figure Q17.1: M-mode echo of the aortic root and left atrium.

ANSWER 17.1. The correct answer is 2, subvalvular aortic stenosis. Figure A17.1 is a magnified view of the aortic valve that shows normal initial opening quickly followed by abrupt partial closure (arrow). This is highly suggestive of subaortic obstruction.

In valvular aortic stenosis and low cardiac output, the aortic valve will not open fully initially. Also, in elderly patients the aortic valve is usually calcified in aortic stenosis. In supravalvular aortic obstruction there will not be early systolic closure of the valve. In subaortic obstruction, the aortic valve opens normally initially, however the high-velocity jet that reaches the valve from the subaortic obstruction creates a lower pressure (Bernoulli or Venturi), which results in partial valve closure.

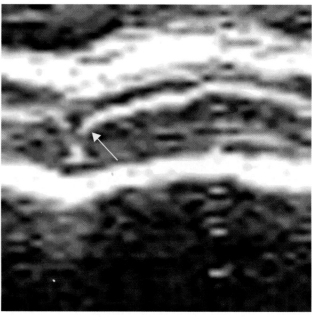

Figure A17.1: Magnified M-mode view of the aortic valve.

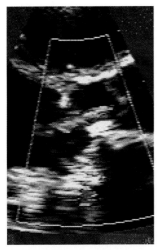

Figure Q17.2B: Same as Figure Q17.2A, diastolic frame, with color.

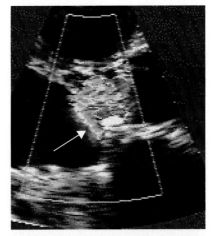

Figure Q17.2C: Same as Figure Q17.2A, systolic frame, with color.

QUESTION 17.2. Figures Q17.2A through Q17.2C are transthoracic 2-D images of this patient. What is the cause of this patient's left ventricular outflow (subaortic) obstruction?

1. Shone's syndrome
2. Hypertrophic obstructive cardiomyopathy
3. Left ventricular outflow tract (LVOT) obstruction by the prosthetic valve
4. Subaortic tunnel

QUESTION 17.3. To further evaluate this patient, calculation of the membrane orifice area was attempted.

Figure Q17.3 shows the apical five-chamber view. The membrane is seen in the left panel (arrows). The proximal isovelocity surface area (PISA) is seen on the color Doppler frame on the right (arrow). The PISA radius is 0.75 cm, and the aliasing velocity is 88 cm/second. The maximal flow velocity on continuous wave Doppler through the membrane was 3 m/second. What is the membrane orifice area?

1. More information is needed
2. 1 cm^2
3. 0.5 cm^2
4. 0.25 cm^2

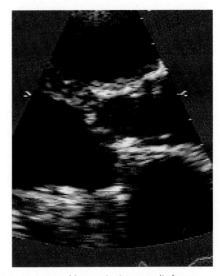

Figure Q17.2A: Parasternal long-axis view, systolic frame.

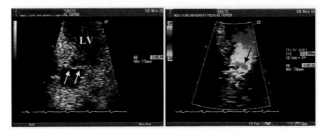

Figure Q17.3. Apical five-chamber views.

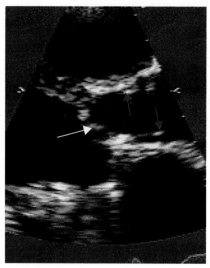

Figure A17.2: Same as Q17.2A.

ANSWER 17.2. The correct answer is 1, Shone's syndrome. This patient had mitral stenosis due to a parachute mitral valve. She also had a subaortic membrane causing LVOT obstruction, which was undiagnosed prior to surgery. These are often present together in Shone's syndrome (along with aortic stenosis, supravalvular membranes and aortic coarctation).

In Figure A17.2, the white arrow points to the subaortic membrane and the red arrows point to the open aortic valve leaflets. The location of the aortic valve closure can be seen on the color Doppler of mild aortic regurtitation (AR) seen in Figure Q17.2B. Note that the origin of the AR jet is about 1 cm above the membrane. Figure Q17.2C shows the high-velocity aliased, turbulent systolic jet that starts at the membrane orifice and fills the LVOT. Just proximal to the membrane one can see proximal isovelocity flow acceleration (arrow).

ANSWER 17.3. The correct answer is 2, 1 cm². The formula used to calculate the membrane orifice area is seen below where Va is the aliasing velocity and Vmax is the maximal velocity through the membrane (Figure Q17.3).

$$\text{Membrane Orifice Area (MOA)} = \frac{2\pi r^2 \times Va}{V\max}$$

$$\text{MOA} = \frac{2 \times 3.14 \times (0.75)^2 \times 88}{300} = 1.05\ \text{cm}^2$$

TAKE-HOME LESSON:

1. **Not every mitral stenosis is rheumatic.**
2. **The subaortic membrane was missed in this patient, who underwent both preoperative echocardiography and cardiac catheterization. A thorough echocardiographic or hemodynamic evaluation would have made the diagnosis.**
3. **Membrane orifice area can be calculated using the PISA technique.**

18 Transient Ischemic Attack Following Myocardial Infarction

*T*hree days after an acute anteroseptal infarction, this 57-year-old man complained of transient difficulty speaking and right-arm weakness. The symptoms resolved in 3 hours. An echo was obtained.

QUESTION 18.1. The echo (Figure Q18.1) showed that there was an apical infarction with an akinetic apex and apical septum, To further evaluate the reason for this patient's symptoms you would do which of the following?

1. Transesophageal echocardiography (TEE)
2. Intravenous (IV) echo-contrast injection
3. Left ventricular (LV) angiography
4. Carotid duplex

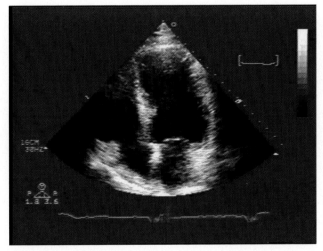

Figure Q18.1: Apical four-chamber view.

ANSWER 18.1. The correct answer is 2, IV echo-contrast injection. Three days after an anteroseptal infarction, the incidence of apical clot is 20%. Although both TEE and carotid duplex scanning may be very valuable in patients with suspected cerebral embolism, the first step should be repeating the echo with contrast. Left ventricular angiography is contraindicated before ruling out an intracavitary thrombus (Figure A18.1).

Note the 2.5-cm filling defect, representing a large apical LV thrombus, which was not visible without the use of contrast.

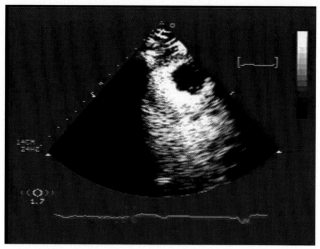

Figure A18.1: Apical view after intravenous echo contrast (Definity).

TAKE-HOME LESSON:

Apical clots may be missed on transthoracic echo. In addition, TEE does not improve visualization of the LV apex.

19 Heart Murmurs

T his patient has had heart murmurs for as long as anyone can remember (Figures Q19.1A and Q19.1B).

QUESTION 19.1. The patient has:

1. Two parents who are frogs
2. Partial atrioventricular (AV) canal
3. Complete AV canal
4. Double inlet left ventricle

QUESTION 19.2. The patient has mitral regurgitation. Which of the following must be true of this patient?

1. He is cyanotic
2. He has exercise intolerance
3. He has a family history of congenital heart disease
4. None of the above

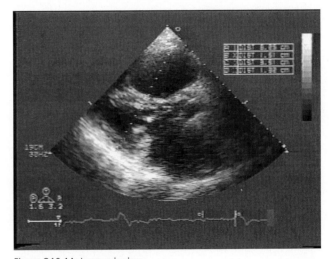

Figure Q19.1A: Long-axis view.

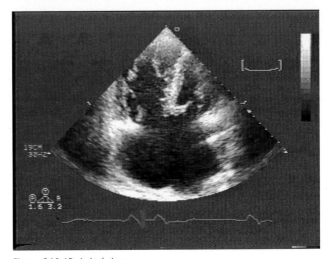

Figure Q19.1B: Apical view.

ANSWER 19.1. The correct answer is 2, partial AV canal. In the parasternal long-axis view (Figure A19.1A), note that the anterior mitral leaflet does not insert at its normal position (arrow). This is a characteristic finding in endocardial cushion defect, because the normal insertion site of the mitral valve is absent. Endocardial cushion defect is a congenital disorder in which structures at the center of the heart do not fuse. It may include ostium primum atrial septal defect (ASD), ventricular septal defect, and cleft mitral valve. Figure A19.1B shows a cleft in the anterior mitral leaflet (arrow). Figure Q19.1B shows the lack of an interatrial septum. Note that there is no interatrial septum at the level of the atrioventricular valves. This defines the ASD as an ostium primum ASD. There is also no septum secundum. This patient does not have a ventricular septal defect, therefore the patient does not have total AV canal. The constellation of findings is known as partial AV canal.

Endocardial cushion defect may be associated with Down's syndrome and congenital rubella.

The patient is not a frog because he is a 73-year-old lawyer. A frog would have two atria and one ventricle, not two ventricles and one atrium.

The patient does not have double inlet left ventricle because there is one atrioventricular valve for each ventricle.

ANSWER 19.2. Correct answer: 4, none of the above.

This patient appears to have a single atrium but in fact there are two atria with no interatrial septum. The pressure in the left atrium is higher than the right atrial pressure throughout the cardiac cycle-in diastole because the left ventricular end-diastolic pressure (LVEDP) is higher than the right ventricular end-diastolic pressure (RVEDP) as with normals and in systole due to mitral regurgitation. Therefore flow mostly occurs from left atrium to right atrium and the patient is NOT cyanotic. Room air oxygen saturation was 95%.

Furthermore, even though he has tricuspid and mitral regurgitation, he is completely asymptomatic. The patient did jumping jacks in the echo laboratory to impress the staff!

The family history may be positive, but not necessarily.

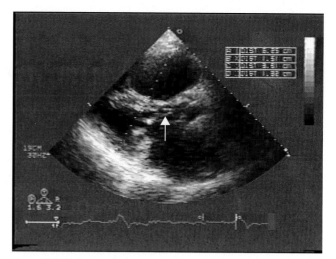

Figure A19.1A: Long-axis view.

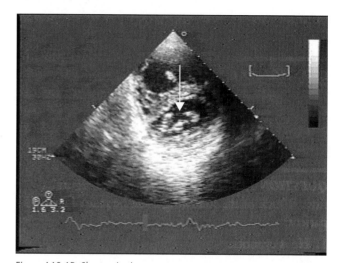

Figure A19.1B: Short-axis view.

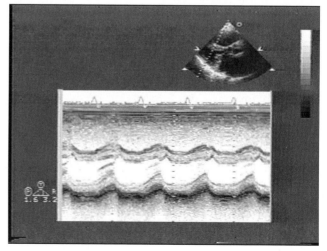

Figure A19.1C: M-mode echo.

How Big Is the Left Atrium?

*A*n 82-year-old woman is admitted with chest pain, and an echocardiogram is done (Figures Q20.1A and Q20.1B).

QUESTION 20.1 How big is the left atrium (LA)?

1. 1 cm
2. 4 cm
3. 6 cm
4. 8 cm

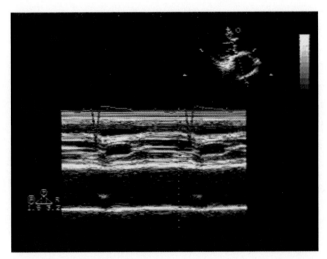

Figure Q20.1A: M-mode echo.

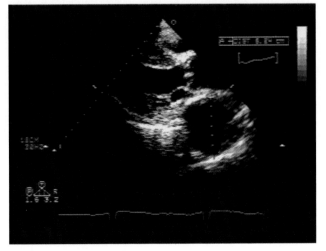

Figure Q20.1B: Long-axis view.

QUESTION 20.2. Figures Q20.2A and Q20.2B are two apical views. The next step for this patient should be

1. Watchful waiting
2. Biopsy
3. Vascular surgery
4. Repair of hiatus hernia
5. Resection of cor triatriatum membrane

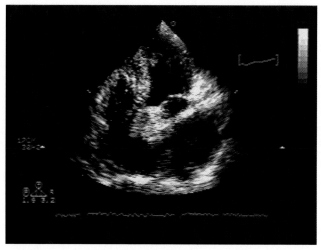

Figure Q20.2A: Apical four-chamber view.

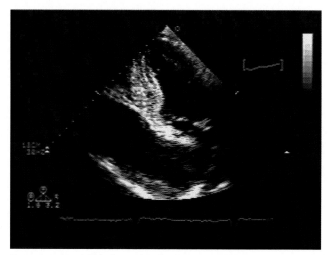

Figure Q20.2B: Modified two-chamber view.

ANSWER 20.1. Correct answer: 1, 1 cm. The left atrium (arrow, Figure A20.1) is compressed externally by a 6-cm mass (asterisk, Figure A20.1).

The M mode is misleading because it doesn't cut through the LA.

ANSWER 20.2. Correct answer: 3, vascular surgery. Figure Q20.2B shows that the mass is a large tubular structure (Figure A20.2). Its location was obtained with backward tilting of the transducer (at the apex). At this site, the descending thoracic aorta is best visualized. This is a large descending aortic aneurysm. Because the patient is symptomatic, surgery is required (resection or stenting). Watchful waiting, or even worse, biopsy, may be life threatening. Although a hiatus hernia may compress the LA, it is not tubular. When in doubt, have the patient drink a carbonated beverage, and echogenic bubbles will appear in the stomach. In this case, a Doppler examination would confirm that the structure has arterial flow. This is not cor triatriatum because the structure extends posterior to the left ventricle.

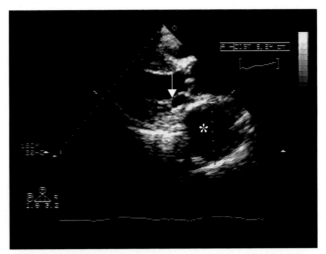

Figure A20.1: Same as Figure Q20.1A.

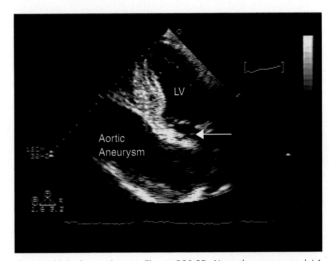

Figure A20.2: Same view as Figure Q20.2B. Note the compressed LA (arrow).

21 Postoperative Transthoracic Echocardiogram

*F*igure Q21.1 was obtained in a 57-year-old female patient in the recovery room after surgery. Her blood pressure (left radial arterial line) was 85/40 mm Hg.

QUESTION 21.1. This echo shows:

1. A pericardial effusion
2. A pleural effusion
3. A vascular abnormality
4. Both 1 and 2 are correct
5. Both 2 and 3 are correct

QUESTION 21.2. To further evaluate this patient's hypotension, you should now:

1. Insert a Swan–Ganz catheter to measure the right ventricular pressure and cardiac output
2. Give an intravenous bolus of 500 ml of saline
3. Measure the blood pressure after evacuation of the pleural effusion
4. Measure the blood pressure in the right arm

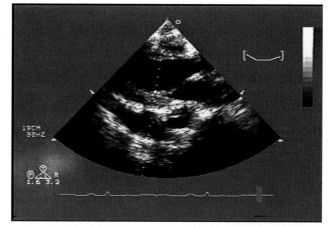

Figure Q21.1: Long-axis view.

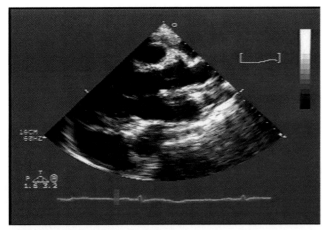

Figure Q21.3A: Long-axis view of the aortic root.

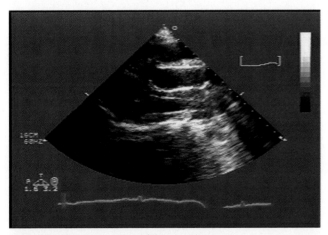

Figure Q21.3B: Long-axis view of the ascending aorta.

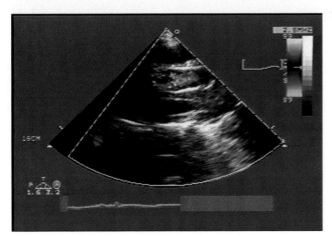

Figure Q21.3C: Same view as Q21.3B, with color flow Doppler. There was no aortic insufficiency.

QUESTION 21.3. Figures Q21.3A, Q21.3B, and Q21.3C show the aortic root and the ascending aorta in this patient.

The patient is asymptomatic. What should you do now?

1. Leave her alone
2. Do an emergency repair of the ascending aortic dissection
3. Operate on the descending aorta and the subclavian artery
4. Put a stent in the descending aorta

ANSWER 21.1. Correct answer: 5, both 2 and 3 are correct. The round structure is the descending thoracic aorta. The line within it (arrow, Figure A21.1A) is suggestive of an intimal (dissection) flap. The echo-free space behind both the left ventricle (LV) and the descending aorta is a pleural effusion (a pericardial effusion will not appear posterior to the descending aorta because the descending aorta is extrapericardial).

Figure A21.1B is a zoomed view, showing the dissection flap.

Although these figures do suggest a dissection flap in the descending aorta, the diagnosis can be more clearly shown by turning the echo transducer 90 degrees to obtain a long-axis view of the descending aorta (Figure A21.1C), which clearly shows that the flap extends parallel to the walls of the descending aorta.

Figure A21.1D shows that the higher velocity blood flow is limited to the true lumen.

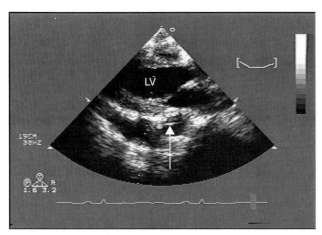

Figure A21.1A: Same view as Figure Q 21.1.

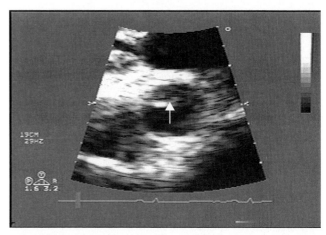

Figure A21.1B: Zoomed long-axis view.

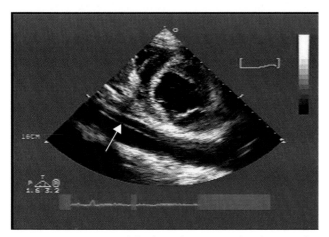

Figure A21.1C: Long-axis of the descending aorta, with a dissection flap within (arrow).

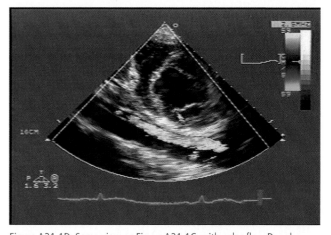

Figure A21.1D: Same view as Figure A21.1C, with color flow Doppler.

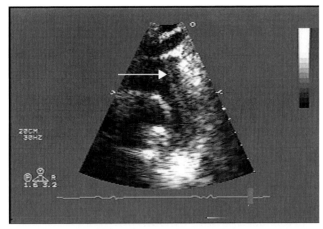

Figure A21.2A: Aortic arch and descending aorta, suprasternal view, with dissection flap within (arrow).

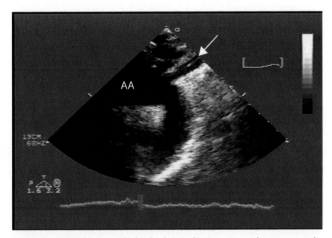

Figure A21.2B: Aortic arch (AA), descending aorta, and great vessels, suprasternal view. Note the dissection flap within the subclavian artery (arrow).

ANSWER 21.2. Correct answer: 4, measure the blood pressure in the right arm. Although the other answers may yield information in patients with hypotension, in a patient with a dissection of the thoracic aorta there may be compromised flow to any of the aortic branches. This could produce a low pressure in the left subclavian artery, but not a low pressure centrally. This patient's blood pressure in the right arm was 140/85 mm Hg. Figures A21.2A and A21.2B show that the dissection flap in the aortic arch (Figure A21.2A) extends into the left subclavian artery (Figure A21.2B).

ANSWER 21.3. The correct answer is 1, leave her alone. This patient had a Type A aortic dissection (which extended from the ascending aorta to the descending aorta). The surgery was limited to the ascending aorta. Figures Q21.3A, Q21.3B, and Q21.3C show that there is a graft in the ascending aorta, with the native aorta wrapped around the graft. The space between the graft and the native aorta is clotted, as expected after this type of repair of an ascending dissection. The residual dissection flap in the arch and the descending aorta is usually left unrepaired. In this patient, the flap in the subclavian artery caused only an asymptomatic compromise in left arm flow, and is better left unrepaired.

TAKE-HOME LESSON:

Although a transesophageal echocardiogram is considered by many to the be diagnostic technique of choice in the evaluation of aortic dissection, in many patients the entire aorta may be visualized by transthoracic echocardiography. These transthoracic views may not be the standard echocardiographic ones, and they should be used in patients with suspected aortic pathology.

22 A 48-Year-Old Man With Fever and Cough

A 48-year-old man was previously well, when he presented with a 3-month history of fever, malaise, and cough. He had seen several physicians, who were treating him for pneumonia. Because of murmurs heard on physical examination, he was referred for transesophageal echocardiography (TEE) to rule out endocarditis (Figures Q22.1A through Q22.1D).

QUESTION 22.1. The aortic valve abnormality most likely represents:

1. Fibroelastoma
2. Myxomatous degeneration with severe aortic valve prolapse
3. Aortic dissection flap prolapsing through the aortic valve
4. Aortic valve aneurysms
5. None of the above

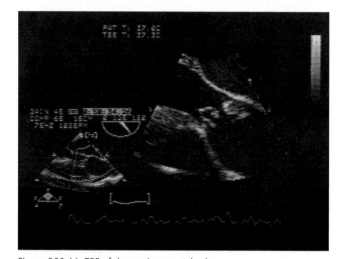

Figure Q22.1A: TEE of the aortic root and valve.

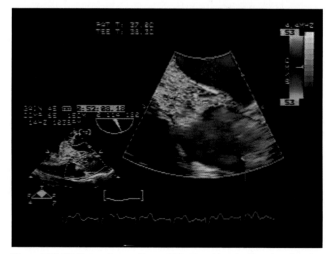

Figure Q22.1B: Same view as Figure Q22.1A, with color Doppler, showing severe AR.

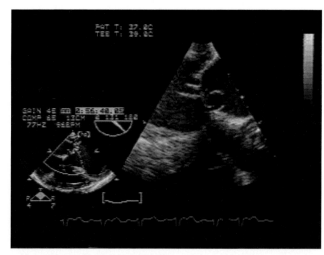

Figure Q22.1C: TEE of the mitral valve.

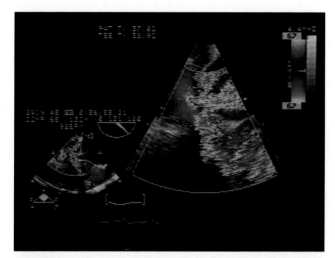

Figure Q22.1D: Same view as Figure Q22.1C, with color Doppler.

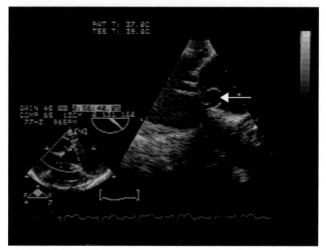

Figure A22.1: Same view as Figure Q22.1C.

QUESTION 22.2. The etiology for the mitral valve abnormality most likely is

1. Myxomatous degeneration
2. Aortic regurgitation (AR)
3. Systemic lupus erythematosus
4. Blood cyst

ANSWERS 22.1 AND 22.2. The correct answers to these two questions are, respectively: 4, aortic valve aneurysms; and 2, aortic regurgitation. This patient has endocarditis with resultant aneurysms of both the aortic and mitral valve. The mitral aneurysm has a distinct perforation (arrow in Figure A22.1), which is responsible for most of the mitral regurgitation (MR).

This patient has endocarditis, with the unusual complications of both aortic and mitral valve aneurysms. The aneurysm of the mitral valve was probably caused by infection/inflammation at the site of the aortic regurgitation jet-lesion on the anterior mitral leaflet. The aneurysm perforated, precipitating very severe MR.

Although the etiology of the aortic valve aneurysm is not certain, it is likely that this was caused by weakening of the valve tissue with infection. On the other hand, the large majority of mitral valve aneurysms occur in the setting of aortic insufficiency during endocarditis.

TAKE-HOME LESSON:
Aortic valve endocarditis may be complicated by mitral regurgitation.

23 Shortness of Breath in a Previously Healthy Patient

A 37-year-old obese woman complained of the recent onset of dyspnea on exertion. An echocardiogram was performed (Figure Q23.1).

QUESTION 23.1. What is wrong?

1. The gain setting is too high
2. Rib artifact
3. Mitral prosthetic valve
4. None of the above

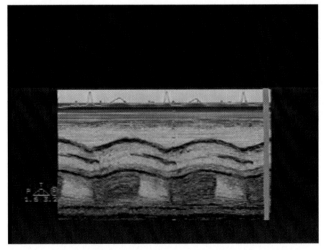

Figure Q23.1: M-mode echo of the aorta and left atrium.

QUESTION 23.2. Review Figures Q23.2A through Q23.2C and decide what is the most likely mass that this patient has.

1. Left atrial (LA) clot
2. LA myxoma
3. LA fibroelastoma
4. No diagnosis can be suggested based on echo alone

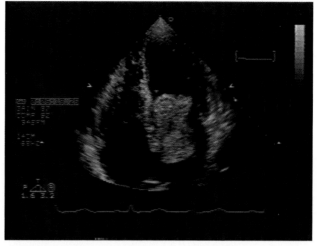

Figure Q23.2A: Apical four-chamber view, diastolic frame.

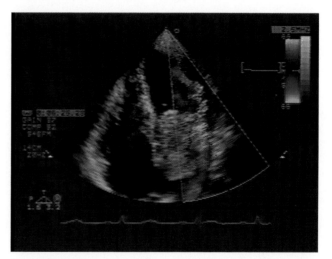

Figure Q23.2B: Same view as Figure Q23.2A, with color Doppler.

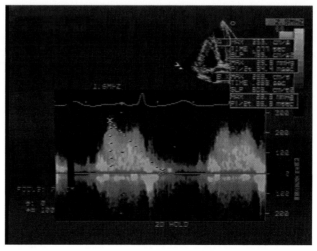

Figure Q23.2C: Continuous wave Doppler through the mitral valve.

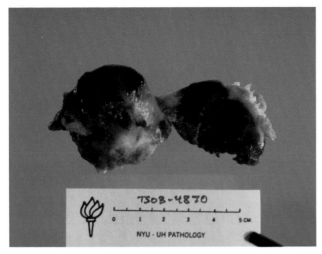

Figure A23.2: Gross pathology of the myxoma.

ANSWER 23.1. Correct answer: 4, none of the above. The gain setting is not too high, as the dark echo shadow only appears in the left atrium during systole. This is not a rib artifact because it only appears in the posterior part of the echo image. The echo from a mitral prosthesis will not appear in the atrium in systole. Thus there is something else causing the echo density in the left atrium.

ANSWER 23.2. Correct answer: 2, LA myxoma. This mass (Figure A23.2) is attached to the interatrial septum, suggesting that this is the most common left atrial tumor, a myxoma. Figure Q23.2C shows that the patient is in normal sinus rhythm, so a clot is very unlikely. Figure Q23.1 shows that the myxoma moves from the left atrium (in systole) into the mitral orifice (in diastole), creating a 20 mm Hg mean gradient across the mitral valve (Figure Q23.2B). This elevation in left atrial pressure is responsible for the patient's dyspnea.

24 Attempt to Record Tricuspid Flow

*T*he following continuous wave (CW) Doppler tracing was obtained in an attempt to record tricuspid blood flow (Figure Q24.1).

QUESTION 24.1. Based on this tracing, which statement is correct?

1. This spectral tracing represents transaortic flow
2. The patient is in shock
3. The patient has hepatomegaly
4. The pulmonary artery (PA) pressure is very low

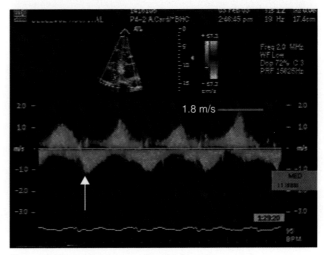

Figure Q24.1: Continuous wave Doppler from the apex.

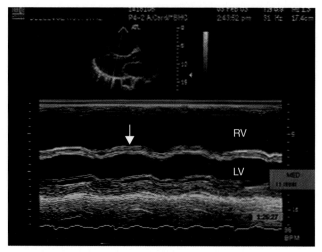

Figure A24.1A: M-mode of the RV and LV.

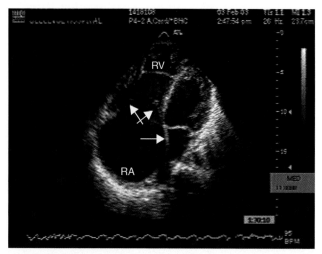

Figure A24.1B: Apical four-chamber view.

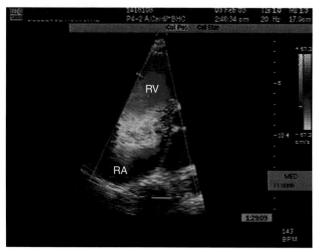

Figure A24.1C: Color Doppler.

ANSWER 24.1. Correct answer: 3, the patient has hepatomegaly. This spectral tracing represents very severe tricuspid regurgitation (TR). There is very little systolic gradient between the right ventricle (RV) and right atrium (RA) (ventricularization of RA pressure). Therefore the TR velocity is only 1 m/second, indicating a maximal gradient of only 4 mm Hg between RV and RA. In late systole, when the pressures equalize, even this small gradient disappears, as seen by the "early peaking" (arrow, Figure Q24.1). In fact, this is a late decline in the velocity. Also, because the TR is very severe, the antegrade diastolic velocity is relatively high (up to 1.8 m/second). Also, the density of the CW tracing is equally high in diastole and systole, because of the large volume of flow.

If this were aortic flow, the spectral tracing of aortic flow would be narrower. Also, if this were aortic flow, one would have to explain the diastolic flow toward the transducer. It is not aortic regurgitation because of the low velocity.

While the patient may be in shock, there is nothing in this tracing to suggest it.

Although the RA pressure is not known, the antegrade flow velocity suggests a large amount of TR (which would be associated with a high RA pressure); therefore while the PA and RA pressures may be similar, they are not necessarily low.

These tracings were obtained in a 27-year-old patient with a history of intravenous drug abuse and tricuspid endocarditis years ago. At the present time, he has right heart failure due to chronic severe TR. The physical examination was remarkable for a holosystolic murmur and a diastolic rumble at the right sternal border, which increased with inspiration. There was also an enlarged liver with systolic pulsation, systolic "CV" waves in the neck veins, and edema.

Note the markedly dilated right ventricle (RV) and paradoxical septal motion (arrow) suggestive of RV volume overload.

Note the markedly enlarged RA and RV in Figure A24.1B. The tricuspid leaflets fail to coapt (small arrows) and the interatrial septum (large arrow) bows toward the left atrium (LA) because the RA pressure is higher than that of the LA.

In Figure A24.1C, note that the TR is low velocity and nonturbulent (blue, with minimal aliasing) because of the large regurgitant orifice and small difference in systolic pressure between the RV and RA.

TAKE-HOME LESSON:

Low-velocity regurgitation is a marker of a very severe lesion (for any valve).

25 What's Wrong With This Mitral Valve?

*A*55-year-old woman has a history of a heart murmur. A continuous wave (CW) Doppler tracing was obtained from the left ventricle (LV) apex (Figure Q25.1).

QUESTION 25.1. What is the physical finding that is most likely to be associated with this Doppler tracing?

1. Diastolic rumble
2. Holosystolic murmur
3. Click
4. Widely split S2

QUESTION 25.2. The degree of severity of this lesion can be best calculated by using:

1. Proximal isovelocity surface area (PISA)
2. Using inflow and outflow volumes for calculation of regurgitant jet volume
3. Color jet area as a percentage of left atrium (LA) area
4. Vena contracta

QUESTION 25.3. Based on Figure Q25.1 (the CW Doppler), the patient should also be treated for:

1. Systemic lupus erythematosus
2. Congestive heart failure
3. Hypertension
4. Atrial septal defect

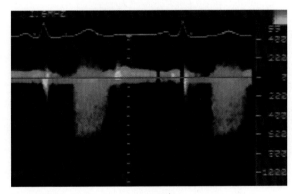

Figure Q25.1: Continuous wave Doppler.

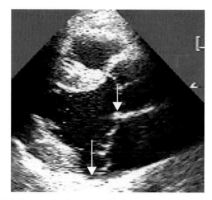

Figure A25.1A: Long-axis view, mitral valve prolapse.

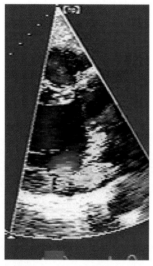

Figure A25.1B: Same view as Figure A25.1A, with color Doppler.

ANSWER 25.1. Correct answer: 3, click. This tracing shows mitral regurgitation due to mitral valve prolapse that is only mid- to end-systolic. The first half of systole (from the QRS to the onset of the T wave) is free of regurgitation. Such an end-systolic murmur is frequently associated with a midsystolic click.

This 2-D long-axis view shows that the mitral leaflets prolapse into the LA, beyond the plane of the mitral annulus (arrows, Figure A25.1A; see also Figure A25.1B).

ANSWER 25.2. Correct answer: 2, using inflow and outflow volumes for calculation of regurgitant jet volume. Answers 1, 2, and 4 all fail to account for the fact that the MR occupies only part of systole, and therefore they will significantly overestimate mitral regurgitation (MR) severity.

To calculate the regurgitant volume, you will have to first measure the left ventricular (LV) inflow volume by multiplying the mitral annulus area by the flow velocity integral of mitral inflow at the mitral annulus. Next, you can calculate the LV forward outflow into the aorta by multiplying the area of the left ventricular outflow tract (LVOT) by the flow velocity integral of the LVOT flow. Because of the mitral regurgitation, the inflow volume is larger than the outflow volume, and the difference between the two represents the mitral regurgitant volume.

ANSWER 25.3. Correct answer: 3, hypertension. The velocity of MR is 6 m/second, and therefore the difference between LV and LA pressures is 144 mm Hg. Even with a normal LA pressure (e.g., 10 mm Hg), the LV pressure (and therefore the aortic pressure) is 154 mm Hg. Although all of the other answers are possible in this patient, there is nothing on the CW tracing that suggests answers 1, 2, or 4.

26 Systolic Aortic Regurgitation

*T*he following systolic frame was obtained from an 80-year-old patient who complained of shortness of breath and palpitations (Figure Q26.1).

QUESTION 26.1. What is malfunctioning?

1. The patient's heart
2. The equipment
3. The sonographer
4. The insurance company

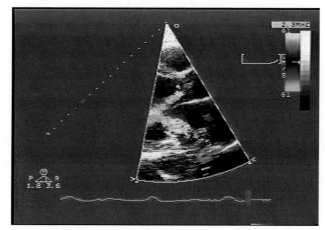

Figure Q26.1: Color Doppler in systole.

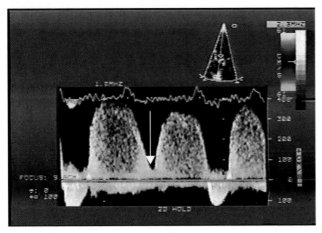

Figure A26.1A: Continuous wave Doppler.

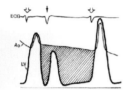

Figure A26.1B: LV and aortic pressures in systolic aortic regurgitation.

ANSWER 26.1. Correct answer: 1, the patient's heart. Figure Q26.1 shows aortic regurgitation occurring at the same time as mitral regurgitation, in systole. Aortic regurgitation may occur normally, during isovolumic relaxation, when aortic pressure is higher than left ventricular (LV) pressure, and the LV declining pressure is still higher than left atrial (LA) pressure. However, this frame is taken later in systole, beyond the isovolumic relaxation period, and has a different mechanism.

The patient is in atrial fibrillation. In the Doppler tracing in Figure A26.1A, after a shorter R-R interval, the systolic pressure produced in the left ventricle is too low to reach aortic pressure and open the aortic valve. Therefore there is no systolic ejection (no antegrade flow below the baseline). The aortic pressure remains higher than the LV pressure throughout the cardiac cycle. All that happens is the velocity of aortic regurgitation diminishes because the LV pressure approaches (but does not exceed) aortic pressure in systole (arrow in Figure A26.1A).

Figure A26.1B shows that with a short R-R interval, LV pressure does not reach the aortic pressure, allowing the pressure gradient between aorta and left ventricle to persist both in systole and diastole (shaded area). This gradient is responsible for aortic regurgitation that occurs both in systole and diastole.

CASE 27 Lobster Claw

*T*his 45-year-old man had an abnormal electrocardiogram (EKG) on a routine insurance examination. With the transducer at the apex, a pulsed Doppler tracing was recorded (Figure Q27.1).

QUESTION 27.1. The tracing in Figure Q27.1 shows:

1. Unidirectional systolic and diastolic flow because of left ventricular (LV) apical hypertrophy
2. Aliased tracing of severe LV outflow obstruction
3. Mitral regurgitation with an incomplete envelope
4. Right-to-left shunting across a small ventricular septal defect

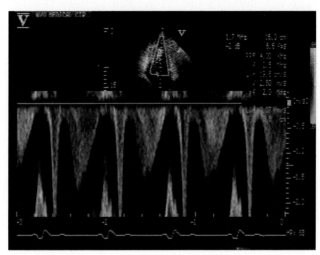

Figure Q27.1: Pulsed wave Doppler from the LV apex.

ANSWER 27.1. Correct answer, 1, unidirectional systolic and diastolic flow because of LV apical hypertrophy. This patient has severe hypertrophy of the LV apex. This is a variant of hypertrophic cardiomyopathy (sometimes associated with giant T waves). There was no LV outflow tract obstruction. The flow pattern seen here was created by obstruction to flow out of the apex in systole, resulting in the short-duration, higher velocity flow (S, Figure A27.1A) seen after the QRS. The duration is short because the diastolic dimension of the hypertrophied LV apical cavity is small, and flow out of this area is small in volume. In spite of that, some blood is trapped in the apex. During diastole, this trapped blood moves in the direction of the LV outflow, producing the diastolic component seen here (D, Figure A27.1A). This pattern looked like a lobster claw

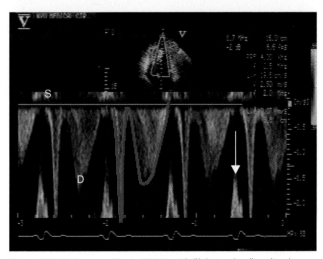

Figure A27.1A: Same as Figure Q27.1, with "lobster claw" outlined.

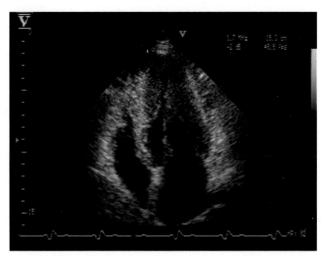

Figure A27.1B: Apical four-chamber view.

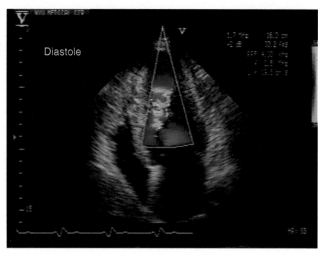

Figure A27.1E: Apical four-chamber view with color Doppler, diastolic frame.

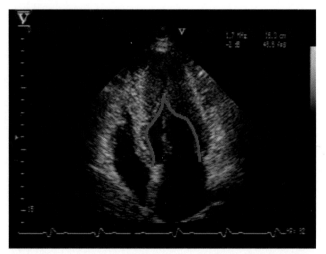

Figure A27.1C: Same as Figure A27.1B, with "spade shape" outlined.

(red outline, Figure A27.1A) to some hungry people. Flow toward the transducer in end-diastole is the A wave of mitral inflow (arrow, Figure A27.1A).

Note the markedly hypertrophied LV apex in Figure A27.1B. The cavity takes on a so-called "spade shape," like the ace of spades (Figure A27.1C).

The blue-green flow is out of the apex in systole (Figure A27.1D).

The red flow represents mitral inflow (Figure A27.1E).

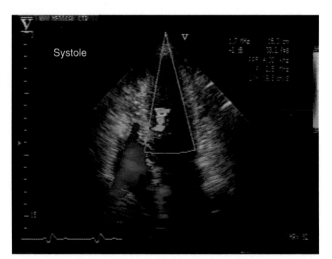

Figure A27.1D: Apical four-chamber view with color Doppler, systolic frame.

28 Chronic Shortness of Breath

*T*his 73-year-old man has been progressively dyspneic for the last 2 years. Physical examination shows edema, hepatomegaly, and distended neck veins. Oxygen saturation on room air is 85%. Transthoracic echo was suboptimal, and a transesophageal echocardiogram was done to rule out intracardiac shunting (Figure Q28.1).

QUESTION 28.1. What is your diagnosis?

1. Pulmonary arterial occlusion
2. Left atrial thrombus
3. Patent ductus arteriosis (PDA) with endocarditis
4. Right ventricular thrombus

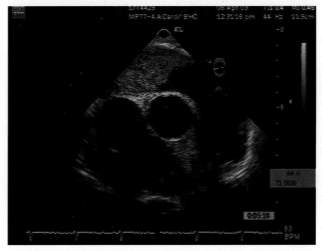

Figure Q28.1: TEE with the transducer angle at 0 degrees.

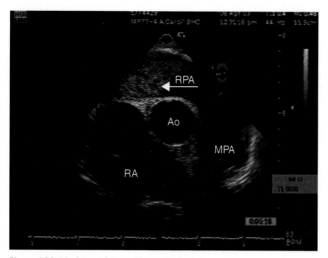

Figure A28.1A: Same view as Figure Q28.1.

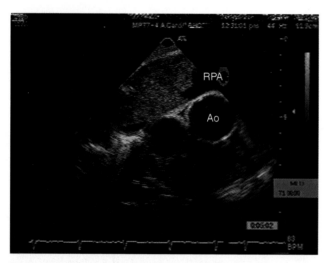

Figure A28.1B. The thrombus extends more distally in the RPA.

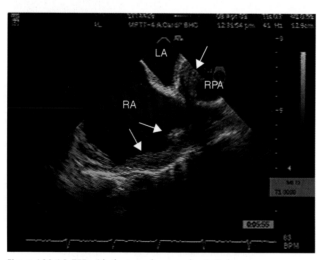

Figure A28.1C: TEE with the transducer angle at 90 degrees.

ANSWER 28.1. Correct answer: 1, pulmonary arterial occlusion. The lumen of the right pulmonary artery is occluded by thrombus (see arrow, Figure A28.1A).

The left atrium (LA) is also a posterior structure; however it is located inferior to the view in Figure A28.1A. The LA does not wrap around the aorta, as does the main pulmonary artery (MPA) and right pulmonary artery (RPA). Usually, left atrial thrombus is seen in a dilated LA, and it is most often in the appendage. A vegetation on the pulmonary arterial side of a PDA can give a mass in the pulmonary artery, but this should be in the left pulmonary artery near the bifurcation (where the PDA enters). The right ventricle is an anterior structure, and can be seen anterior to the aorta (Ao). The right atrium (RA) and MPA are dilated.

Note in Figure A28.1B how the thrombus extends more distally in the RPA.

In the view seen in Figure A28.1C, the right pulmonary artery can be seen just behind the superior vena cava. There is thrombus (arrow pair, Figure A28.1C) in the RA as well as the RPA (single arrow, Figure A28.1C).

TAKE-HOME LESSON:

Proximal pulmonary emboli can be frequently identified on transesophageal echocardiography. Transesophageal echocardiography should be performed in patients with unexplained pulmonary hypertension or dyspnea.

Pleural Effusion and Abnormal Echo

*T*his 29-year-old man was admitted to the hospital with a productive cough and fever. He was treated for pneumonia with improvement in his symptoms. Because of an abnormal cardiac silhouette on x-ray, an echo was performed (Figures Q29.1A and Q29.1B).

QUESTION 29.1. What diagnoses are suggested?

1. Atrial Septal Defect (ASD)
2. Absent pericardium
3. Severe tricuspid regurgitation (TR)
4. Numbers 1 and 3 are correct
5. Numbers 1, 2, and 3 are correct

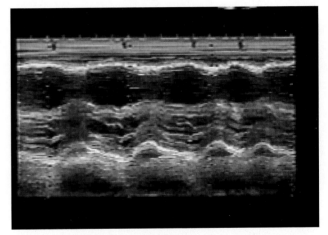

Figure Q29.1A: M-mode echo, parasternal.

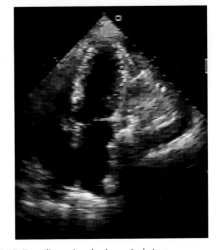

Figure Q29.1B: Two-dimensional echo, apical view.

ANSWER 29.1. Correct answer: 5, numbers 1, 2, and 3 are correct. Figure Q29.1A shows a dilated right ventricle (RV) and paradoxical septal motion. These findings are seen in patients with RV volume overload (present in ASD with a left-to-right shunt, and in patients with severe TR (or pulmonic regurgitation [PR]). However, paradoxical septal motion is also seen in congenital absence of the pericardium (the correct diagnosis in this case). In this entity, there is translation of the heart to the left and anterior motion of the heart in systole. The leftward translation changes the orientation of the RV so that this wedge-shaped structure is cut differently by M-mode echo and appears to be enlarged. The posterior wall motion is also exaggerated, and the septal motion is paradoxical, because the whole heart moves anteriorly in systole with the lack of pericardial restraint. Doppler echo showed no TR or PR, and there was no evidence of ASD.

What is also characteristic of absent pericardium is that the left lung (seen in Figure Q29.1B, with the pleural effusion, which is due to this patient's pneumonia) is in direct contact with the left ventricle (LV).

TAKE-HOME LESSON:

Right ventricular dilatation and paradoxical septal motion is frequently due to RV volume overload, but don't forget the rare patient with absent pericardium. While this condition may be post-surgical, a rare patient may have it from birth (partial, or complete as in this patient).

30 Oxygen Desaturation

*T*his 38-year-old man was admitted with dyspnea. Oxygen desaturation (88%) was noted. A spectral Doppler tracing was obtained during transesophageal echocardiography (Figure Q30.1).

QUESTION 30.1. Based on this tracing, the patient's desaturation is a result of:

1. Mitral stenosis
2. Left ventricular (LV) outflow obstruction
3. Pulmonic stenosis (PS) with patent ductus arteriosus (PDA)
4. Right-to-left shunt

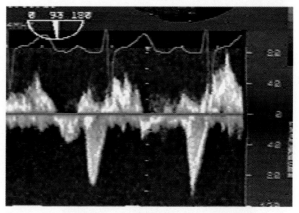

Figure Q30.1: Pulsed wave Doppler during TEE, 90-degree view.

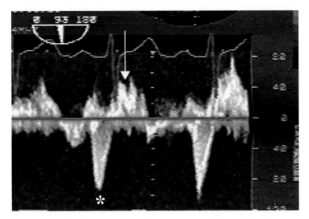

Figure A30.1A. Same view as Figure Q30.1.

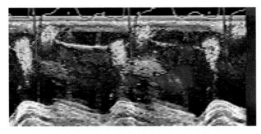

Figure A30.1B: Color M-mode. Note the left-to-right shunt in blue-green, and the right-to-left shunt in red.

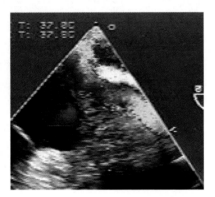

Figure A30.1C: Two-dimensional echo, TEE, systolic frame. Note the right-to-left shunt in red.

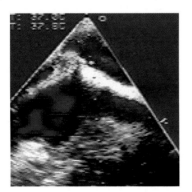

Figure A30.1D: Two-dimensional echo, TEE, end-diastolic frame. Note the left-to-right shunt in blue/aliased to orange.

ANSWER 30.1. Correct answer: 4, right-to-left shunt. There is a bidirectional shunt across an atrial septal defect. Low-velocity flow toward the transducer is noted in systole (arrow, Figure A30.1A), and there is also flow away from the transducer (asterisk, Figure A30.1A) at end-diastole, with atrial contraction. The study does not suggest mitral stenosis because the diastolic flow velocity is only approximately 1 m/second and the diastolic flow (asterisk, Figure A30.1A) does not have the appearance of the jet seen in mitral stenosis (in which it is holodiastolic, with an increased pressure half-time and slow flow deceleration). There is no LV outflow obstruction because the systolic velocity noted here is low (approximately 60 cm/second). Finally, if the patient had PS and a PDA, there would be only left-to-right shunting because of the low pulmonary artery (PA) pressure (also there is nothing on this tracing to suggest PS).

Color Doppler (Figures A30.1B, A30.1C, and A30.1D) clearly demonstrates bidirectional shunting.

This patient has a small-to-moderate sized atrial septal defect. He now suffers from an increase in PA pressure secondary to pulmonary embolization. In ventricular systole, the pressure is higher in the right atrium than in the left atrium and there is right-to-left shunting. With atrial contraction, the opposite is true and there is left-to-right shunting.

> *TAKE-HOME LESSON:*
> **Although there are many reasons for oxygen desaturation, one should always consider the possibility of a right-to-left intracardiac shunt.**

31 Why Is This Young Woman Short of Breath?

*F*or the last 2 years, this 22-year-old woman has been increasingly short of breath and unable to walk uphill and climb stairs. Her father died at the age of 27. Physical examination revealed an S4 gallop, but was otherwise unremarkable. Her electrocardiogram (EKG) showed nonspecific T-wave changes, and her chest x-ray was unremarkable. An echocardiogram was ordered (Figures Q31.1A and Q31.B).

The left ventricular ejection fraction was normal. There was no significant valvular pathology.

QUESTION 31.1. The diagnosis is

1. Noncompaction of the ventricles
2. Hypertrophic cardiomyopathy (nonbstructive)
3. Rhabdomyoma
4. Amyloidosis
5. Agent Orange poisoning

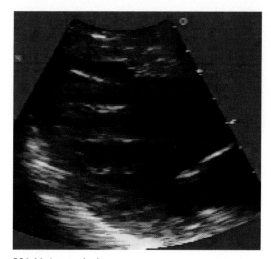

Figure Q31.1A: Long-axis view.

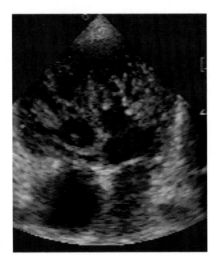

Figure Q31.1B: Apical four-chamber view.

QUESTION 31.2. The transmitral flow pattern in this patient will most likely show:

1. E = 60 cm/second; A = 130 cm/second; deceleration time = 220 msec; e' (tissue Doppler) = 10 cm/second
2. E = 120 cm/second; A = 120 cm/second; deceleration time = 220 msec; e' = 12 cm/second
3. E = 170 cm/second; A = 30 cm/second; deceleration time = 100 msec.; e' = 12 cm/second.
4. E = 170 cm/second; A = 30 cm/second; deceleration = 100 msec; e' = 4 cm/second

ANSWER 31.1. Correct answer: 1, noncompaction of the ventricles. Note that both ventricles have very marked trabeculation. This is due to an embryonic developmental abnormality, in this case involving both ventricles (it may also be limited to the left ventricle). The disorder is associated with heart failure, arrhythmia, and intracardiac clot formation with embolization. Rhabdomyoma would produce a localized mass. In hypertrophic cardiomyopathy, the wall(s) will be thick but compacted, without dramatically excessive trabeculation. Amyloidosis may produce thickening of the wall(s), but they will be compacted normally. Finally, although Figure Q31.1A is orange, Agent Orange has not been reported to produce this change in the echocardiogram.

ANSWER 31.2. Correct answer: 4, E = 170 cm/second; A = 30 cm/second; deceleration = 100 msec; e' = 4 cm/second This patient has symptoms of a markedly elevated LA pressure in spite of a normal ejection fraction and no mitral valve disease. This is consistent with diastolic dysfunction. Therefore the mitral E velocity is high (170), the A velocity is low (30), the deceleration time is very short (100 msec; normal > 160 msec). All of these findings may be seen in restrictive or constrictive disease. However, the tissue Doppler shows a low e' velocity. The E : e' ratio is markedly elevated (43). This is therefore characteristic of restrictive myocardial disease, in this case caused by noncompaction. In constrictive pericarditis, tissue Doppler e' will be normal.

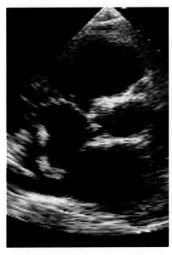

CASE 32 Chest Pain

A 62-year-old man has a history of three myocardial infarctions. He now presents with chest pain and dyspnea. A transthoracic echocardiogram recently showed an ejection fraction of 20%. A repeat echo is ordered (Figures Q32.1A through Q32.1C).

QUESTION 32.1. What was the predisposing factor in this case?

1. Congestive heart failure
2. His recent plane trip from Santo Domingo
3. Factor V Leiden
4. All of the above

QUESTION 32.2. The mobile mass in the right atrium (RA) is most likely which of the following?

1. Clot
2. Pacemaker wire
3. Papillary fibroelastoma
4. Chiari network

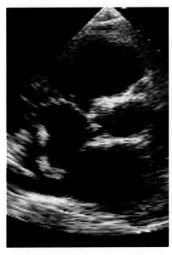
Figure Q32.1B: Another short-axis view.

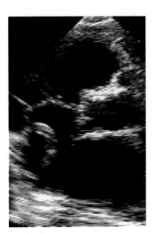
Figure Q32.1A : Short-axis view.

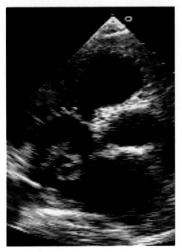
Figure Q32.1C: A third short-axis view.

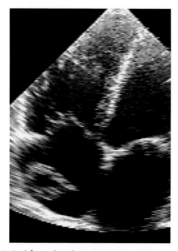

Figure A32.2: Subxiphoid view.

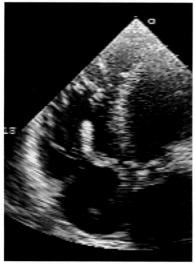

Figure A32.3A: Apical four-chamber view.

Figure A32.3B: Apical four-chamber view.

ANSWER 32.1. Correct answer: 4, all of the above.

ANSWER 32.2. Correct answer:1, clot. This is a long, worm-like, serpiginous structure that is a cast of the leg veins. A pacing wire is more echogenic and thinner. Papillary fibroelastoma is typically round or oval, and may have finger-like projections. A Chiari network is a normal fetal membrane that extends from the inferior vena cava (IVC) to the opening of the coronary sinus. It serves to direct blood from the lower body across the atrial septum during fetal life, and can remain as a "rest" in adults.

The patient has a deep vein thrombosis in his leg, and has embolized clot from the ilio-femoral venous system to his right atrium, and to his lungs. The clot is highly mobile, as can be seen from its varying appearances in Figures Q32.1A through Q32.1C. Figure A32.2 shows the inferior vena cava.

Note the clot in the IVC just at its juncture with the RA. The IVC is dilated (> 2.5 cm) and does not collapse with inspiration ("IVC plethora").

There was mild tricuspid regurgitation. The velocity of the tricuspid regurgitation was 3.5 m/second.

QUESTION 32.3. What is the estimated pulmonary artery (PA) systolic pressure? The tricuspid regurgitation (TR) velocity is 3.5 m/second.

1. 50 mm Hg
2. 30 mm Hg
3. Over 70 mm Hg
4. It can not be calculated from the available data

ANSWER 32.3. Correct answer: 3, over 70 mm Hg. The patient's RA pressure can be estimated as > 20 mm Hg because there is IVC plethora. The right ventricular-right atrial (RV–RA) systolic gradient is 50 mm Hg (the velocity of the TR is 3.5 m/second, therefore the RV–RA systolic gradient is $4V^2$, or 50 mm Hg). The PA systolic pressure equals this gradient plus the RA pressure.

Note that the clot is moving through the tricuspid valve (in diastole) (Figures A32.3A and A32.B).

Because of his pulmonary hypertension and dilated, hypokinetic right ventricle, thrombolysis was considered. However it was felt to be contraindicated because of the patient's gross hemoptysis (which may occur more often in patients with pulmonary infarction who have high left-heart diastolic pressures). Surgery was also felt to be very high risk. The patient was treated with intravenous heparin and recovered.

33 Echo After Invasive Procedure

A 49-year-old man recently underwent an invasive cardiac procedure. The following echo was obtained with the patient on the catheterization table (Figures Q33.1A through Q33.1G).

QUESTION 33.1. This study shows which of the following?

1. Ostium Primum atrial septal defect (ASD)
2. Ostium Secundum ASD
3. Sinus Venosus ASD
4. None of the above

QUESTION 33.2. The contrast injection was made into which of the following?

1. The pulmonary artery
2. The left basilar vein
3. The inferior vena cava
4. The right lower pulmonary vein

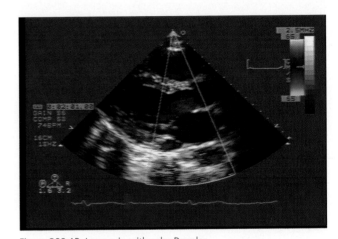

Figure Q33.1B: Long axis, with color Doppler.

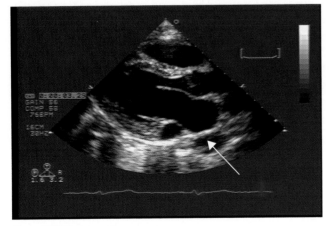

Figure Q33.1A: Long axis.

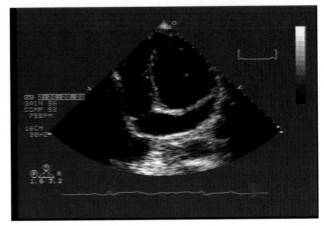

Figure Q33.1C: Apical view.

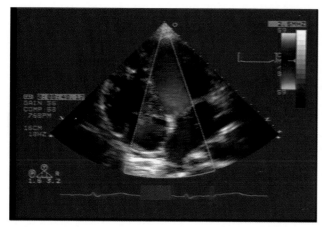

Figure Q33.1D: Four-chamber view.

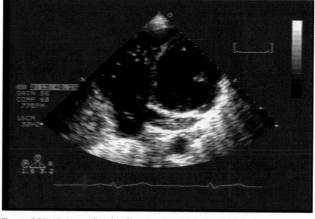

Figure Q33.1F: Immediately after IV agitated saline injection.

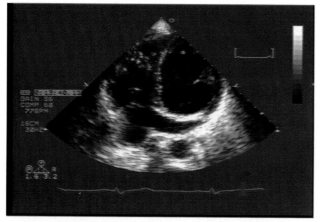

Figure Q33.1E: Before intravenous (IV) agitated saline injection.

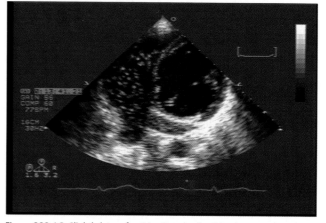

Figure Q33.1G: Slightly later after IV agitated saline injection.

QUESTION 33.3. The structure marked with an arrow in Figure Q33.1A is which of the following?

1. The coronary sinus
2. The descending aorta
3. A renal cyst
4. A paracardiac abscess

ANSWER 33.1. The study shows a dilated coronary sinus. The answer is 4, none of the above. The interatrial septum is intact, as seen in Figure Q33.1D. Tilting the transducer backward may create the impression that there is an interatrial communication (see Figure Q33.1C); however, this is the dilated coronary sinus entering the right atrium posterior to the interatrial septum.

ANSWER 33.2. The correct answer is 2, the left basilic vein. This patient has a persistent left superior vena cava that is

connected to the coronary sinus (which is therefore dilated). After left arm injection, microbubbles first appear in the dilated coronary sinus (Figure Q33.1F), and then they appear in the right atrium and right ventricle (Figure Q33.1G). Agitated saline injection into the pulmonary artery will be trapped in the lungs. Injection into the inferior vena cava will appear directly in the right atrium (and not first in the coronary sinus, which is connected to the *left* superior vena cava). The right lower pulmonary vein normally is connected to the left atrium. If it is anomalous, it may be directly connected to the right atrium (not through the coronary sinus).

ANSWER 33.3. The structure marked with an arrow in Figure Q33.1A is 2, the descending aorta, which normally appears in this position on the long-axis view. The coronary sinus is seen within the pericardium (the aorta is not). A renal cyst and a paracardiac abscess will not have blood flow as seen in Figure Q33.1B.

The invasive procedure was ablation (of paroxysmal atrial flutter). During the procedure, the coronary sinus was noted to be dilated, and this prompted the echo.

34 Cardiogenic Shock

*T*hree years after aortic valve replacement, this 45-year-old woman presented with severe chest pain and hypotension. On physical examination, her blood pressure was 70/50, the chest was clear, and there was marked jugular venous distention. Transthoracic echo showed good left ventricular (LV) function, normal mechanical aortic valve function, and a dilated right ventricle. The international normalized ratio (INR) was 2.1. Transesophageal echocardiography (TEE) was performed (Figure Q34.1).

Note the dilated right ventricle (RV) and right atrium (RA). The RV was almost akinetic.

QUESTION 34.1. What is your diagnosis?

1. Constrictive pericarditis
2. Aortic valve clot
3. Cardiac tamponade
4. Acute myocardial infarction (MI)
5. 1 and 3 are correct
6. 2 and 4 are correct

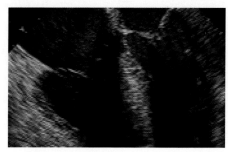

Figure Q34.1: TEE four-chamber view.

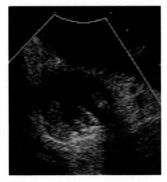

Figure A34.1: TEE of the St. Jude's aortic prosthesis.

ANSWER 34.1. Correct answer: 6, both 2 and 4 are correct (aortic valve clot and acute MI).

This patient had thrombosis of a St. Jude's aortic prosthesis with embolization to the right coronary artery and right ventricular infarction. The clot formation did not interfere with normal prosthetic valve function.

Note in Figure A34.1 that there is a clot within the prosthesis, in the anterior portion of the aorta near where the right coronary orifice would be.

The patient underwent coronary angiography that revealed total occlusion of the right coronary artery by a clot. The other coronary arteries were normal. Angioplasty and stenting restored right coronary artery flow, and there was marked hemodynamic improvement.

TAKE-HOME LESSON:
Prosthetic valve clots do not necessarily result in valve stenosis or insufficiency, but they definitely can embolize. The INR should be kept between 2.5 and 3.5 in patients with mechanical prostheses.

35 Postoperative Echo

*T*his 38-year-old man had surgery 6 years ago. Review Figures Q35.1A through Q35.1I and try to decipher the following:

QUESTION 35.1. What are the patient's symptoms?

1. Cyanosis
2. Pulmonary edema
3. Ankle edema
4. Facial edema

QUESTION 35.2. What was the surgery 6 years ago?

1. Tricuspid repair
2. Mitral repair
3. Glenn procedure
4. Mustard procedure

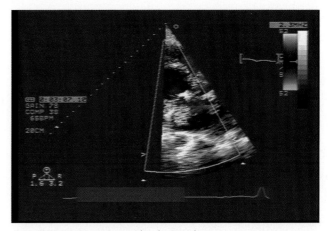

Figure Q35.1B: Same view, with color Doppler.

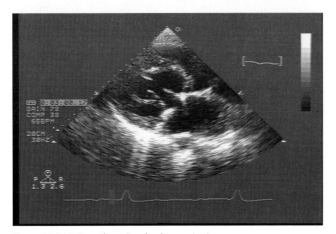

Figure Q35.1A: Transthoracic echo, long-axis view.

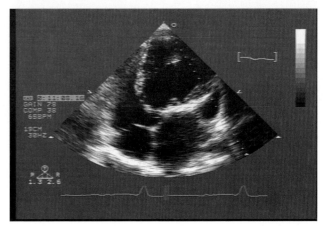

Figure Q35.1C: Apical view.

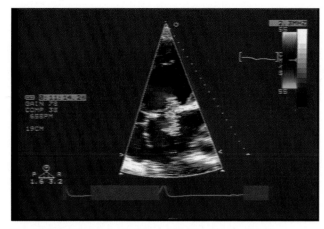

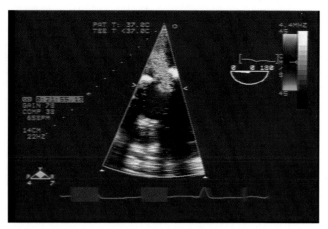

Figure Q35.1D: Same view as Figure Q35.1C, with color Doppler.

Figure Q35.1G: Same TEE view, with color Doppler.

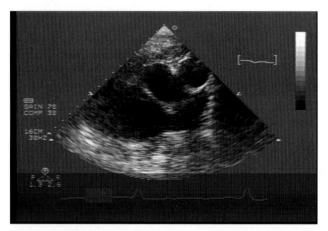

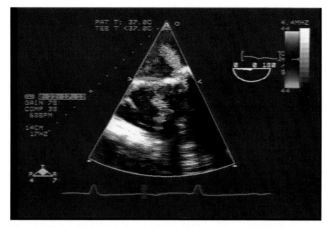

Figure Q35.1E: Short-axis view, base of the heart.

Figure Q35.1H: Same TEE view, wider angle.

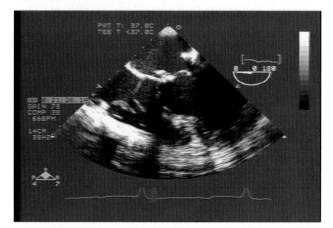

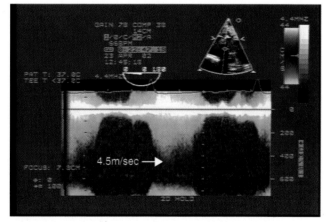

Figure Q35.1F: You have probably solved it by now, but for addition information, here is the TEE. TEE, four-chamber view, zero degrees.

Figure Q35.1I: Same view, CW Doppler.

QUESTION 35.3. This study also shows which of the following?

1. atrial septal defect (ASD)
2. ventricular septal defect (VSD)
3. patent ductus arteriosis (PDA)
4. Surgically repaired D transposition

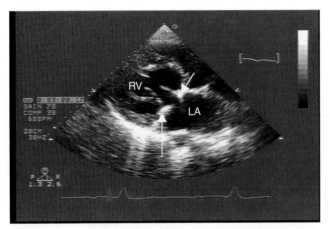

Figure A35.1A: Same as Figure Q35.1A.

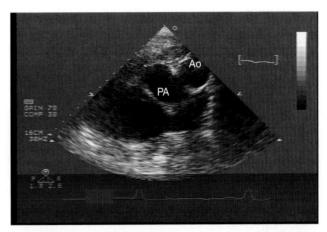

Figure A35.1C: Same as Figure Q35.1E.

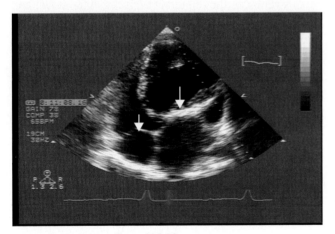

Figure A35.1B: Same as Figure Q35.1C.

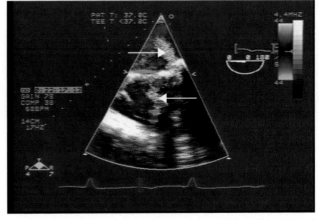

Figure A35.1D: Same as Figure Q35.1H. Note the VSD jet (lower arrow) and the TR (upper arrow).

ANSWER 35.1. The patient's symptoms were most likely to be 2, pulmonary edema.

ANSWER 35.2. The surgery 6 years ago was 1, a tricuspid repair, with a Carpentier ring.

ANSWER 35.3. This study also shows 2, a VSD.

This patient has congenitally corrected transposition of the great vessels, L transposition. In such a patient, the aorta is contiguous with the anatomic right ventricle (RV) and the pulmonary artery is contiguous with the anatomic left ventricle (LV). However, the ventricles are also transposed, and therefore the circulation is "corrected." The left atrium is connected to the right ventricle (now the systemic ventricle), which empties into the aorta. The right atrium is connected to the left ventricle (the venous ventricle), which empties into the pulmonary artery. Thus the pulmonary venous flow ends up in the aorta, and the systemic venous flow ends up in the pulmonary artery, as it should. Because the valves always remain in their correct anatomic ventricles, the tricuspid valve is in the right ventricle (in these patients, the systemic ventricle), and the mitral valve is in the left ventricle (in these patients, the venous ventricle).

Patients with L transposition frequently develop failure of both the anatomic right ventricle and its tricuspid valve, because neither of these is designed to deal with the systemic pressures. The result of failure of the systemic ventricle and its valve (the anatomic RV and tricuspid valve) is elevation of the left atrial pressure and pulmonary congestion.

Our patient suffered from pulmonary edema, and underwent tricuspid valve repair (Figure Q35.1A). As seen in Figure A35.1A, there is a tricuspid ring in place (arrows). Note that in Figure A35.1A the ventricle is not connected to the aorta via an outflow tract because this is not the LV, it is the anatomic RV.

Unfortunately, the tricuspid repair failed, and there is significant tricuspid regurgitation (TR) seen in Figures Q35.1B, Q35.1D, and Q35.1G. This resulted in pulmonary edema and led to a second tricuspid valve repair.

The apical four-chamber view (Figure Q35.1C) and the transesophageal echocardiogram (TEE) four-chamber view (Figure Q35.1F) show yet another diagnostic feature: The tricuspid valve is situated closer to the ventricular apex than is the mitral valve (as it is normally). This allows you to diagnose the fact that the right repair is to the tricuspid valve. However, because there is ventricular inversion, the regurgitation is from the RV into the left atrium (LA).

Note that in Figure A35.1B the longer arrow points to the tricuspid valve (closer to the RV apex), and the smaller arrow points to the mitral valve (farther from the LV apex).

In addition, the two great vessels are transposed. In Figure A35.1C, they are seen side by side, with the pulmonary artery (PA) slightly posterior to the aorta (Ao) and coursing posteriorly.

The TEE also shows an additional finding, namely a VSD. This is seen in Figure A35.1D.

The VSD velocity is high, 4.5 m/second, as seen in Figure Q35.1I.

For those who wonder about the other options for answers:

This patient would not have cyanosis. The shunt is from the higher pressure systemic ventricle to the lower pressure venous ventricle. He is also unlikely to have any signs of right heart failure such as ankle edema, since the high-velocity VSD jet indicates a low PA pressure. There is no reason for facial edema, which would be seen in superior vena cava syndrome or after a Glenn procedure (see next paragraph).

The surgical repair was not a mitral repair (the valve in the venous ventricle, the anatomic LV, is the mitral valve, and appears to be normal). A Glenn procedure is a connection that is made between the SVC and the right pulmonary artery. It is done in patients with a hypoplastic right heart (tricuspid atresia and/or pulmonic atresia) not applicable here. Although the great vessels are transposed, this was corrected congenitally by ventricular inversion. There was no need to do a Mustard procedure (which is done in patients with uncorrected, D transposition). In this procedure a baffle is put in place of the atrial septum to divert systemic venous blood into the anatomic left ventricle, and pulmonary venous blood into the anatomic right ventricle in a patient with D transposition.

TAKE-HOME LESSON:
Congenital heart disease can be quite complex, and can later be complicated by acquired problems.

CASE

36 Rheumatic Heart Disease

A 72-year-old woman had severe progressive exertional dyspnea. This Doppler echocardiogram was done to provide a hemodynamic evaluation (Figures Q36.1A through Q36.1K). At the time of the echo the blood pressure (BP) was 110/80.

QUESTION 36.1. What is the pulmonary artery (PA) pressure (in mm Hg)?

1. Cannot calculate without measurement of the right atrial (RA) pressure
2. About 50/10
3. About 70/30
4. About the same as the systemic BP (110/80)

QUESTION 36.2. What is the left ventricular (LV) pressure (in mm Hg)?

1. 95/27
2. 158/16
3. 180/16
4. 210/36

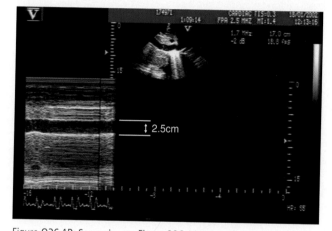

Figure Q36.1B: Same view as Figure Q36.1A, M-mode.

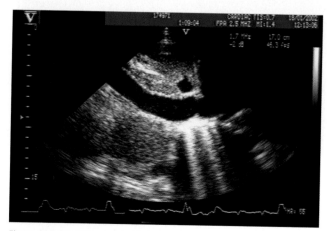

Figure Q36.1A: IVC, subxiphoid view.

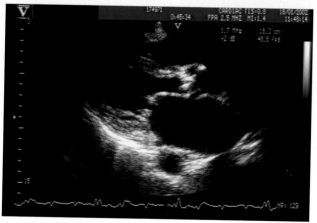

Figure Q36.1C: Long-axis view.

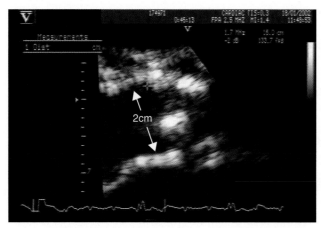

Figure Q36.1D: Same view as Figure Q36.1C, with LVOT zoomed.

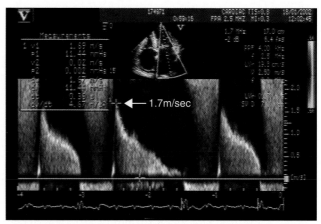

Figure Q36.1G: Apical four-chamber view, CW of transmitral flow.

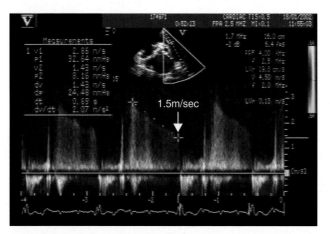

Figure Q36.1E: Short-axis view, CW of pulmonic regurgitation.

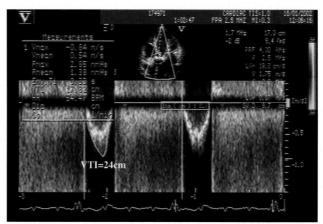

Figure Q36.1H: Apical long-axis view, pulsed Doppler of LVOT.

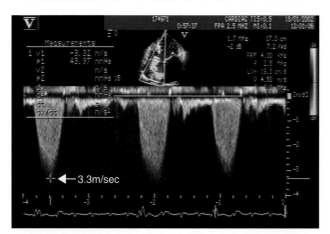

Figure Q36.1F: Apical four-chamber view, CW of tricuspid regurgitation.

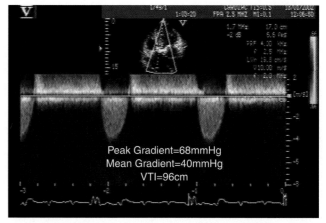

Figure Q36.1I: Apical five-chamber view, CW of aortic stenosis.

QUESTION 36.3. What is the aortic valve area (in cm2)?

1. About 0.4
2. About 0.8
3. About 1.2
4. About 1.4

QUESTION 36.4. What is the severity of the mitral stenosis (MS)?

1. Mild
2. Moderate
3. Severe
4. Cannot be calculated in the presence of significant mitral regurgitation (MR)

QUESTION 36.5. Because of her symptoms, surgery was considered. What would you recommend?

1. Mitral and aortic valve replacement
2. Mitral repair and aortic replacement
3. Triple valve replacement (tricuspid, mitral, and aortic)
4. Tricuspid repair, mitral and aortic valve replacement

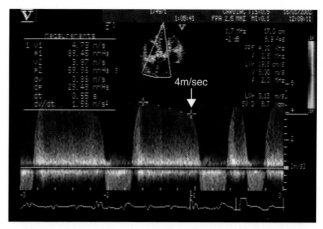

Figure Q36.1J: Same view as Figure Q36.1I, CW of aortic insufficiency.

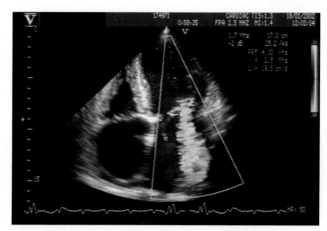

Figure Q36.1K: Apical four-chamber view, with color Doppler.

ANSWER 36.1. The correct answer is 3, the PA pressure is about 70/30 mm Hg. The right atrial pressure can be estimated from the inferior vena cava (IVC) size and its lack of collapse with inspiration. The RA pressure is therefore at least 20 mm Hg. The tricuspid regurgitation velocity is 3.3 m/second, indicating a gradient of 44 mm Hg in systole between the RV and the RA. Therefore the PA systolic pressure is at least 20 plus 44 (about 70 mm Hg). The PA diastolic pressure is equal to the gradient between the PA and the RV, plus the RV diastolic pressure (which in the absence of TS is equal to the RA diastolic pressure, or 20 mm Hg). The pulmonic regurgitation (PR) end-diastolic velocity is 1.5 m/second, indicating an end-diastolic gradient of 9 mm Hg between the PA and RV. Thus, the PA diastolic pressure is approximately 30 mm Hg (9 + 20).

ANSWER 36.2. The correct LV pressure is 2, 158/16. The peak instantaneous systolic gradient across the aortic valve is 68 mm Hg. The peak-to-peak gradient is lower, approximately 70% of the peak instantaneous gradient, or 48 mm Hg. Because the systolic BP is 110, the peak LV systolic pressure is 110 + 48, or 158 mm Hg. From the continuous wave (CW) Doppler of aortic regurgitation, you can see that the end-diastolic velocity is 4 m/second. Therefore the end-diastolic gradient between the aorta and the LV is 64 mm Hg and the LV end-diastolic pressure equals the diastolic systemic BP (80 mm Hg) minus this gradient (64 mm Hg). The LV end-diastolic pressure is therefore 16 mm Hg.

ANSWER 36.3. The correct answer for the aortic valve area is 2, about 0.8 cm^2. This is obtained using the continuity equation:

$A_2 \times VTI_2 = A_1 \times VTI_1$, where A_2 is the aortic valve area, VTI_2 is the time velocity integral of transaortic flow (96 cm), A_1 is the LVOT area (if the diameter is 2 cm, the LVOT area is 3.14 cm^2), and VTI_1 is the time velocity integral of the LVOT flow as measured by pulsed Doppler (24 cm). Thus, A_2 (the aortic valve area) equals 3.14 × 24 / 96, or approximately 0.8 cm^2.

ANSWER 36.4. The severity of MS is 1, mild. Although the peak velocity of transmitral flow in diastole is 1.7 m/second, the mean velocity is much lower and the pressure half-time slope is short.

ANSWER 36.5. The correct operation for this patient would be 4, tricuspid valve repair and replacement of the aortic and mitral valves. The mitral valve is rheumatic, thickened, and (mildly) stenotic. Results of repair for such valves are suboptimal, and the valve has to be replaced because of the severe MR (as seen in Figure Q36.1K).

TAKE-HOME LESSON:
Most hemodynamic data may be obtained non-invasively using Doppler echocardiography. This eliminates the need for cardiac catheterization in the evaluation of most patients with valvular heart disease.

37 Abnormal Blood Count

*T*his patient with fever was referred for echo to rule out endocarditis (Figures Q371A through Q37.1D). The complete blood count (CBC) showed a markedly elevated white blood count.

QUESTION 37.1. No vegetations were seen. Can you offer a diagnosis?

1. Endocarditis
2. Tuberculosis
3. Chronic pericarditis
4. Chronic myelogenous leukemia

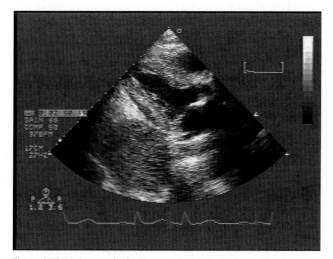

Figure Q37.1A: Long-axis view.

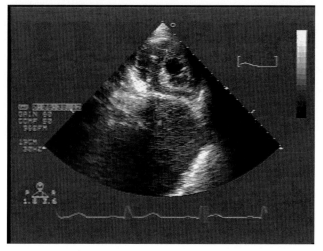

Figure Q37.1B: Short-axis view.

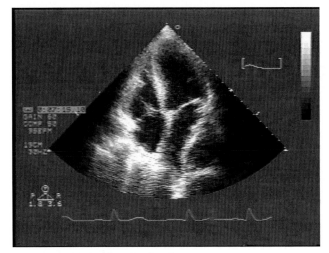

Figure Q37.1C: Apical four-chamber view.

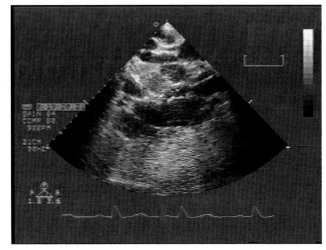

Figure Q37.1D: Modified short-axis view, at the base of the heart.

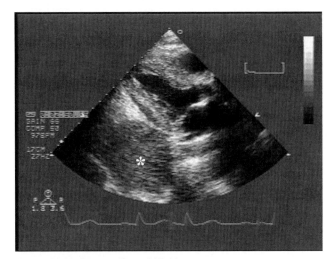

Figure A37.1A: Same as Figure Q37.1A.

ANSWER 37.1. Correct answer: 4, chronic myelogenous leukemia. The white blood count was 110,000. Although 25% of patients with native valve endocarditis may have a negative transthoracic echocardiogram (without vegetations), this patient has a huge mass (more than 10 cm) posterior and inferior to the left ventricle (LV) (asterisk, Figure A37.1A).

This mass is the markedly enlarged spleen. In Figure A37.1B, the mass can be seen to deform the posterior wall of the LV (arrow).

In addition, Figure Q37.1D shows enlarged para-aortic lymph nodes.

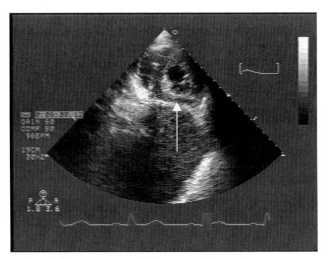

Figure A37.1B: Same as Figure Q37.1B.

C A S E

38 Name This Structure

*T*his 45-year-old man with palpitations had marked cardiomegaly on chest x-ray.

QUESTION 38.1. What is this structure (*) in Figure Q38.1?

1. Left atrial appendage (LAA)
2. Aneurysm of the descending aorta
3. Extracardiac mass
4. Dilated coronary sinus

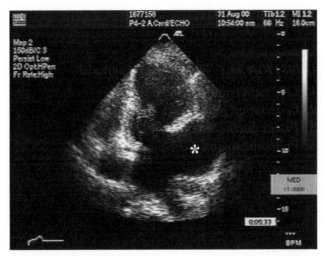

Figure Q38.1: Transthoracic echocardiogram, apical four-chamber view.

ANSWER 38.1. Correct answer: 1, left atrial appendage. This patient has a huge congenital aneurysm of the left atrial appendage, as confirmed on a transesophageal echocardiogram (TEE) (Figure A38.1).

Note that the LAA is contiguous with the body of the left atrium (LA).

The descending aorta was normal, and the "mass" is clearly part of the heart. The coronary sinus drains into the right atrium (RA), not the LA (except in very rare cases of "unroofing" of the coronary sinus). Even in cases of persistent left-superior vena cava, the coronary sinus is not this dilated.

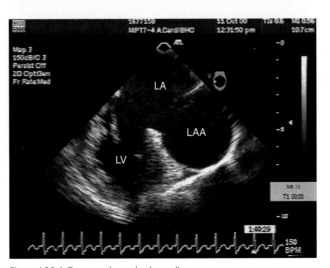

Figure A38.1: Transesophageal echocardiogram.

39 Heart Murmur in an Elderly Patient

*T*his 82-year-old woman is scheduled for on-pump coronary bypass surgery. A preoperative evaluation revealed a heart murmur, and an echocardiogram was ordered (Figures Q39.1A and Q39.1B).

QUESTION 39.1. What is your diagnosis?

1. Left main coronary artery stenosis
2. Coarctation of the aorta
3. Patent ductus arteriosus (PDA)
4. Pulmonic stenosis

QUESTION 39.2. Now that you have established the diagnosis, what is your advice to the surgeon who is doing the coronary bypass operation?

1. Just do the coronary artery bypass graft (CABG), and ignore the PDA
2. Cancel the operation, it is too complicated
3. Deal with the other lesion first, and then do the CABG
4. Do the CABG first, and then deal with the other lesion

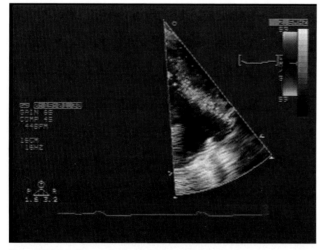

Figure Q39.1A: Short-axis view, at the base of the heart.

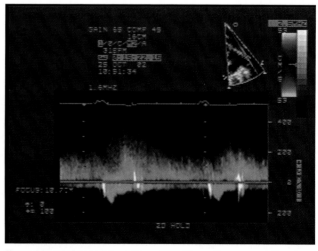

Figure Q39.1B: Same view as Figure Q39.1A, continuous wave Doppler.

ANSWER 39.1. Correct answer: 3, PDA.

In Figure A39.1A, note the turbulent, high-velocity flow emanating from the left pulmonary artery (L); (R = right pulmonary artery, M = main pulmonary artery). This is the characteristic site of entry of the communication between the aorta and the pulmonary artery in PDA.

Figure Q39.1B shows that the flow toward the transducer is continuous (systolic and diastolic), which reaches its peak at end-systole, around the second heart sound. This creates the characteristic machinery murmur. The origin, the direction, and the velocity of the flow rule out stenosis of the left main coronary artery. The antegrade velocity across the pulmonic valve is normal, and therefore there is no pulmonic stenosis.

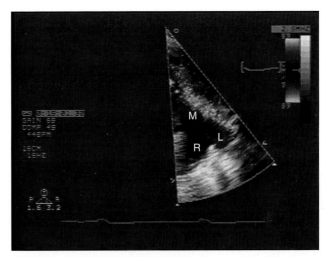

Figure A39.1A: Same view as Figure Q39.1A.

ANSWER 39.2. Correct answer: 3, deal with the PDA (the other lesion) first; otherwise it will be difficult to go on full cardiopulmonary bypass because some of the blood entering the aorta will return to the left heart via the PDA and the lungs. The PDA can either be ligated, or occluded before the surgery with coils (percutaneously). Care must be taken with ligation, as the PDA may be calcified in this elderly patient.

TAKE-HOME LESSON:

You are never too old to have congenital heart disease.

40 Dyspnea in a Patient With Lymphoma

*T*his 68-year-old man is receiving chemotherapy for non-Hodgkin's lymphoma. The transesophageal echocardiogram (TEE) (Figures Q40.1A and Q40.1B) was ordered because of increasing dyspnea with pleuritic chest pain and vague findings on the transthoracic echo.

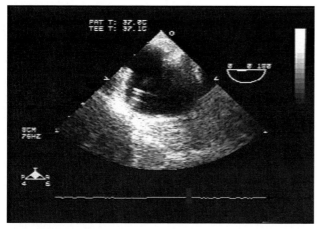

Figure Q40.1A: Transesophageal echocardiogram, 0-degree view, at the level of the RA.

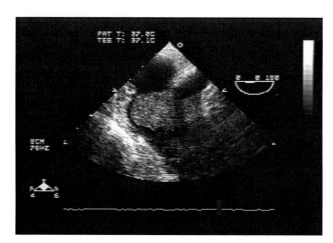

Figure Q40.1B: Same view as Figure Q40.1A, another frame.

QUESTION 40.1. What is the diagnosis?

1. Right atrial lymphoma
2. Iatrogenic complication
3. Right atrial myxoma
4. Artifact

ANSWER 40.1. Correct answer: 2, iatrogenic complication. This patient has a mediport catheter, which has migrated into the right atrium (RA) (arrow, Figure A40.1A). The bright echo appearance is characteristic of a catheter or wire.

A huge, mobile clot has formed on the catheter, as seen in Figure A40.1B. A slightly different cut exposes both the catheter and the clot

Additional workup revealed multiple pulmonary emboli, which were causing the patient's dyspnea.

TAKE-HOME LESSON:

The position of such catheters should be checked to ensure that they have not migrated. Even in the vena cava, thrombosis is possible.

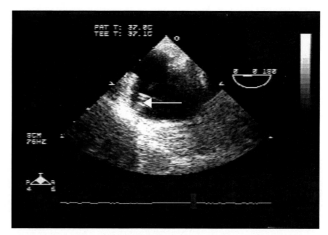

Figure A40.1A: Same view as Figure Q40.1A.

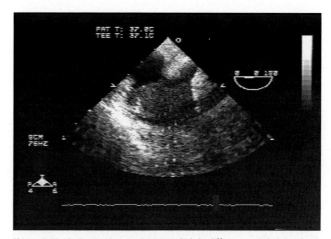

Figure A40.1B: Same view as Q40.1B, slightly different cut showing both the clot and the catheter within it.

CASE 41 Hypertension

A 16-year-old girl was referred for transthoracic echocardiography for the evaluation of hypertension (Figures Q41.1A and Q41.B).

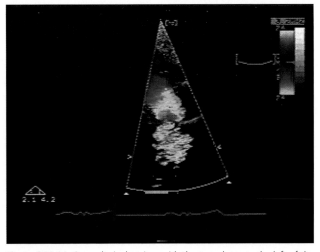

Figure Q41.1A: Supraclavicular view with the transducer to the left of the sternal notch.

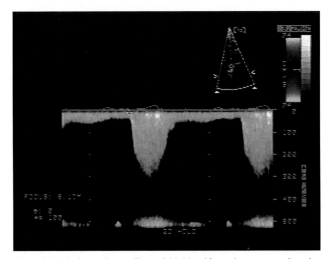

Figure Q41.1B: Same view as Figure Q41.1A, with continuous wave Doppler.

QUESTION 41.1. What is your diagnosis?

1. Aortic stenosis
2. Supravalvular aortic stenosis
3. Subvalvular aortic stenosis
4. Aortic coarctation

QUESTION 41.2. The operator needs to know the cross-sectional area of the stenosis. How will you determine this?

1. magnetic resonance imaging (MRI)
2. computed tomography (CT)
3. transesophageal echocardiogram (TEE)
4. Use the information you already have
5. All of the above

ANSWER 41.1. Correct answer: 4, aortic coarctation. There is a 3-m/second systolic jet going away from the transducer, in the descending aorta. There is a much slower velocity jet in diastole. In all of the other conditions, the jet will be toward the transducer in the supraclavicular window.

Additional workup showed that the patient's blood pressure increased significantly with moderate exertion, and stenting of the coarct was considered.

ANSWER 41.2. Correct answer: 5, all of the above. Although answers 1, 2, and 3 are correct, it is easier (and less expensive) to use the information you already have from the transthoracic echo. Figure A41.2 shows that there is a proximal isovelocity surface area (PISA) visible where blood accelerates toward the coarctation (arrow).

We can use the PISA method to calculate the effective coarctation area (ECA). Using the maximal systolic PISA radius of 1 cm, an aliasing velocity (V_a) of 74 cm/second, and a peak transcoarctation systolic velocity (V_{max}) of 310 cm/second:

$$\text{Effective Coarctation Area (ECA)} = \frac{2\pi R^2 V_a}{V_{max}}$$

$$\text{ECA} = \frac{2 \times 3.14 \times 1^2 \times 74}{310} = 1.5 \text{ cm}^2$$

This patient also underwent MRI, which confirmed the echocardiographic findings.

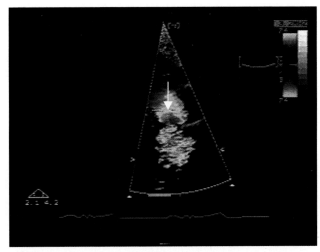

Figure A41.2. Same view as Figure Q41.1A.

TAKE-HOME LESSON:

Although the PISA method is better known for the calculation of the severity of regurgitant lesions, it can also be used to calculate the area of stenotic valvular and other stenotic lesions (such as coarctation).

CASE 42 Name This Syndrome

*T*his 26-year-old man underwent surgery 1 year ago. He now presents with a murmur (Figures Q42.1A through Q42.1E).

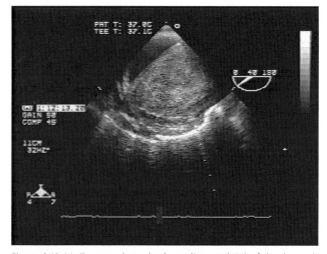

Figure Q42.1A: Transesophageal echocardiogram (TEE) of the descending aorta.

QUESTION 42.1. This patient may also complain of which of the following?

1. Visual disturbances
2. Diarrhea
3. Hot flashes
4. Skin rash on the elbows

QUESTION 42.2. What is the most likely diagnosis?

1. Type-A aortic dissection
2. Suboptimal repair
3. Aortic insufficiency
4. All of the above
5. None of the above

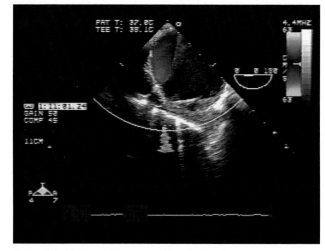

Figure Q42.1B: Descending aorta, with color Doppler.

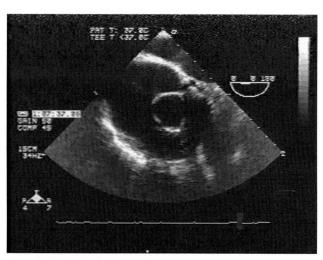

Figure Q42.1C: TEE of the ascending aorta, zero degrees.

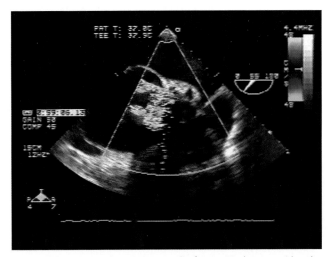

Figure Q42.1D: Ascending aorta, systolic frame, 30 degrees with color Doppler.

Figure Q42.1E: Ascending aorta, diastolic frame, 24 degrees, with color Doppler.

ANSWER 42.1. Correct answer: 1, visual disturbances. The patient has Marfan's syndrome and is s/p repair of Type A aortic dissection. The reason for the visual disturbance is ectopia lentis, another manifestation of Marfan's syndrome.

ANSWER 42.2. Correct answer: 4, all of the above.

Figure Q42.1A shows a markedly dilated descending aorta, with a dissection flap and clot in the false lumen. Figure Q42.1B shows blood flow in the true lumen. Figure Q42.1C shows a huge ascending aorta (7 cm), within which there is a much smaller round graft (3.2 cm). Figure Q42.1D shows that there are two leaks leading from the graft into the ascending aorta (arrows in Figure A42.1A). Therefore the surgical results are definitely suboptimal. These leaks increase the pressure in the wrap of the ascending aorta around the graft, which may lead to rupture, and therefore they have to be repaired. Figure Q42.1E shows that there is aortic regurgitation also (arrow in Figure A42.1B), which is responsible for the patient's murmur.

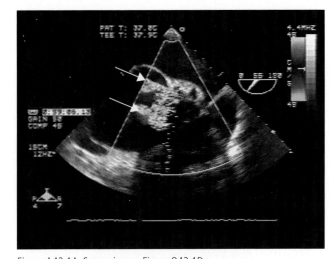

Figure A42.1A: Same view as Figure Q42.1D.

Patients with a Type A dissection (which are dissections involving the ascending aorta) need to have urgent surgical repair. This often includes grafting the ascending aorta, and leaving the native aorta wrapped around the graft. The space between the graft and the wrap usually clots and obliterates (which it did not do in this case because of the two leaks). In this patient, the descending aorta is also markedly dilated. (This is not true in most Marfan's patients, although Marfan's syndrome may involve any part of the aorta, even the abdominal aorta.)

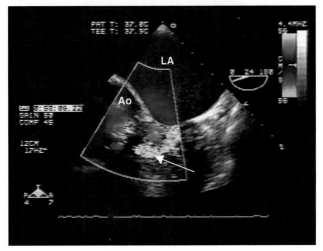

Figure A42.1B: Same view as Figure Q42.1E.

CASE

43 New Murmur

*T*his 28-year-old previously healthy woman was referred for echocardiography because of a new murmur. A previous echo 5 years ago was normal. Figure Q43.1 is a continuous wave Doppler obtained from the subxiphoid view.

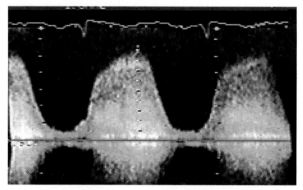

Figure Q43.1: Continuous wave Doppler, subxiphoid view.

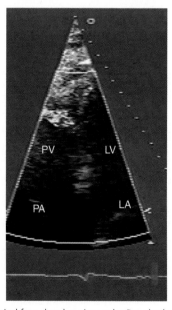

Figure Q43.2: Apical four-chamber view, color Doppler (technically suboptimal, but note the color jet from the left to the right ventricle).

QUESTION 43.1. What is the diagnosis?

1. Mitral regurgitation
2. Tricuspid regurgitation and pulmonary hypertension
3. Ventricular septal defect (VSD)
4. Hypertrophic obstructive cardiomyopathy with outflow tract obstruction
5. Pulmonary infundibular stenosis

QUESTION 43.2. The most likely etiology for the lesion in Figure Q43.2 is

1. Rupture of septal abscess due to endocarditis
2. Rupture of a coronary artery aneurysm
3. Myocardial infarction
4. Stab wound to the chest

ANSWER 43.1. Correct answer: 3, ventricular septal defect. In addition to the high-velocity flow toward the transducer in systole, there is also low-velocity diastolic flow, both in early-diastole and late-diastole (Figure A43.1, arrows).

Although all of the other choices may be associated with high-velocity systolic flow, VSD will usually have diastolic flow also in both early-diastole and late-diastole. This occurs because the left ventricular pressure usually exceeds that in the right ventricle throughout diastole (increasing with the atrial kick in late-diastole, as in Figure A43.1).

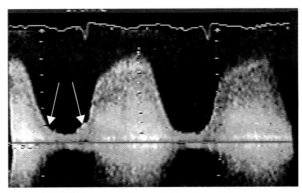

Figure A43.1: Same view as Figure Q43.1.

ANSWER 43.2. Correct answer: 4, stab wound to the chest. In our violent world, a stab wound unfortunately is not a rare occurrence. All of the other entities are rare in 28-year-old patients. This patient's boyfriend stabbed her 15 times in the chest with an ice pick.. She underwent pericardiocentesis in the emergency room for treatment of tamponade. A hole in the right ventricle was sutured and she had an uneventful recovery. The VSD was picked up later because of the murmur. The shunt was small and no treatment (except for antibiotic prophylaxis) was indicated. This represents an "acquired Maladie de Roger."

44 Murmur After Valve Replacement

*T*his 44-year-old woman with a recent mitral valve replacement had an echocardiogram because of a postoperative systolic murmur (Figure Q44.1).

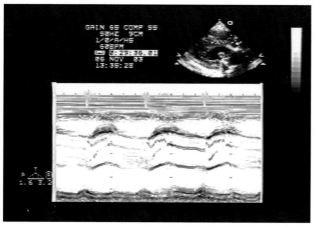

Figure Q44.1: M-mode of the aortic root and left atrium (LA).

QUESTION 44.1. What type of valve was implanted?

1. Carpentier–Edwards tissue prosthesis
2. Bjork–Shiley tilting disk prosthesis
3. St. Jude's medical "bileaflet" disk prosthesis
4. Lillehei–Kaster tilting disk prosthesis

ANSWER 44.1. Correct answer: 1, Carpentier–Edwards tissue prosthesis. The M-mode echo shows that there is early systolic partial closure of the aortic valve, as is seen with subaortic stenosis. This is more commonly seen with hypertrophic obstructive cardiomyopathy, when the mitral systolic anterior motion puts the mitral valve in contact with the interventricular septum, causing left ventricular outflow tract (LVOT) obstruction. It is also seen in patients with membranous subaortic stenosis, when the high-velocity jet that travels through the aortic valve creates an area of lower pressure, resulting in apposition of the aortic leaflets. However, it may rarely be present when a tissue prosthesis (a high-profile valve) is implanted into a relative small left ventricle (as is usually present in patients with mitral stenosis). In this case, a strut of the tissue prosthesis is in contact with the interventricular septum (see Figure A44.1A), causing outflow tract obstruction (see Figure A44.1B). The other answers are all low-profile valves, which do not obstruct the outflow tract.

Note that a strut of the prosthesis is in contact with the septum (arrow) in Figure A44.1A.

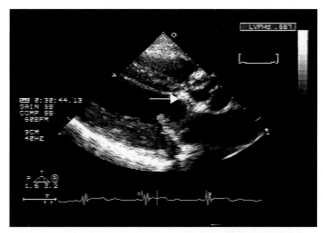

Figure A44.1A: Two-dimensional echocardiogram, long–axis view.

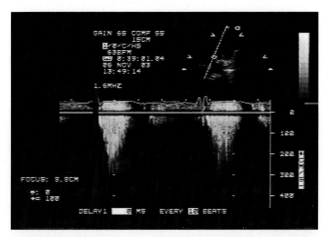

Figure A44.1B: Continuous wave Doppler, showing that there is a 36 mm Hg gradient across the left ventricular outflow tract.

TAKE-HOME LESSON:

A tissue prosthesis (a high-profile valve) may not fit adequately into a relatively small left ventricle, and it may cause LVOT obstruction. Intraoperative transesophageal echocardiography is crucial in order to avoid this problem. Correct orientation of the tissue prosthesis may avoid having contact between the strut and the septum. A low-profile mechanical valve may be necessary if LVOT obstruction is unavoidable.

Murmur After Aortic Valve Replacement

A 66-year-old woman had a mechanical aortic valve replacement (AVR) for aortic stenosis. Because a postoperative murmur was heard, an echocardiogram was performed (Figure Q45.1).

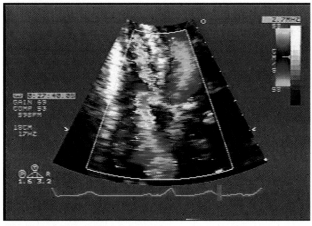

Figure Q45.1: Apical view, color Doppler.

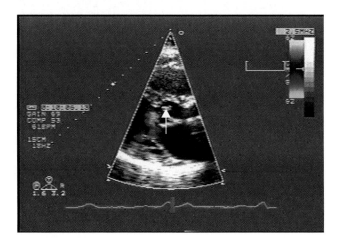

Figure Q45.2: Color Doppler, long-axis view.

QUESTION 45.1. What is the diagnosis?

1. Tricuspid regurgitation (TR)
2. Mitral regurgitation
3. Atrial septal defect
4. Ventricular septal defect (VSD)
5. 1 and 4 are correct
6. 2 and 3 are correct

QUESTION 45.2. What does Figure Q45.2 show (arrow)?

1. Coronary artery flow
2. Eccentric jet of aortic regurgitation
3. Aortic stenosis
4. VSD

QUESTION 45.3. What operation (in addition to the AVR) was done?

1. Mitral valve replacement (MVR)
2. Tricuspid valve replacement (TVR)
3. Dissection repair
4. Septal myomectomy

ANSWER 45.1. Correct answer: 5, both 1 and 4 are correct. Two abnormal color jets are seen in the right heart (Figures A45.1A and A45.1B). The color Doppler (at end-systole) shows both tricuspid regurgitation (in the RA, long arrow) and a turbulent, aliased flow in the right ventricle (RV) (short arrow), which represents a VSD.

ANSWER 45.2. Correct answer: 1, coronary artery flow. This is a coronary-cameral fistula. The amount of shunt resulting is negligible (as opposed to the amount from the VSD).

ANSWER 45.3. Correct answer: 4, septal myomectomy. The myomectomy done to prevent left ventricular outflow tract (LVOT) obstruction after the aortic valve replacement went too far and caused a ventricular septal defect, which was the cause of the murmur. It also amputated a septal perforator, resulting in the coronary artery–cameral (chamber) fistula. This fistula is a not uncommon finding after myomectomy. One would not expect it after answers 1, 2, or 3.

In Figure A45.3, note that the septum has been resected (myomectomy) proximal to the aortic valve (arrow).

TAKE-HOME LESSON:
Septal myomectomy should extend far enough into the left ventricle to reduce LVOT obstruction, but it should not extend into the right ventricle!

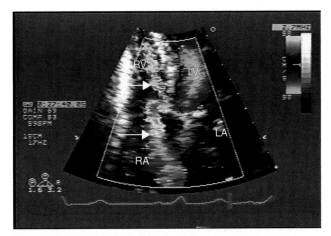
Figure A45.1A: Same view as Figure Q45.1.

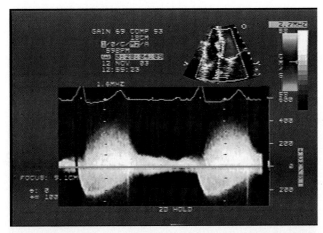
Figure A45.1B: Continuous wave Doppler, showing both the VSD and the TR.

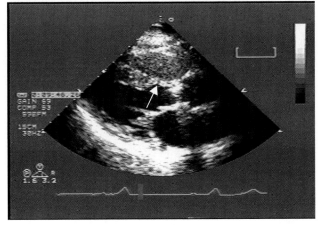
Figure A45.3: Two-dimensional echo, long-axis view.

CASE

46 Unusual Mitral Valve

*T*his 39-year-old man had an echocardiogram because of a heart murmur (Figure Q46.1).

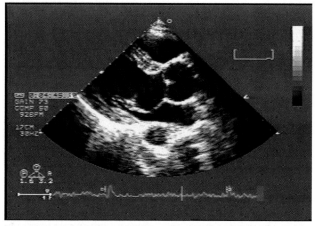

Figure Q46.1: Two-dimensional echo, long-axis view, end-diastolic frame.

QUESTION 46.1. The mitral valve has an unusual appearance. What is the etiology of this patient's heart disease?

1. Rheumatic
2. Traumatic
3. Congenital
4. Infectious

QUESTION 46.2. What is the anatomic diagnosis?

1. Parachute mitral valve
2. Shone's syndrome (multiple obstructions: parachute mitral valve, subaortic membrane, coarctation, etc.)
3. Tetralogy of Fallot
4. Bicuspid aortic valve

ANSWER 46.1. Correct answer: 3, congenital.

ANSWER 46.2. Correct answer: 4, bicuspid aortic valve. In such patients, there is often aortic regurgitation with an eccentric jet directed downward toward the mitral valve. In this patient this has caused restriction in mitral valve opening (note the downward curve in the anterior leaflet).

In Figure A46.2A, note the posteriorly directed jet of aortic regurgitation, which travels along the anterior mitral leaflet.

Note how the mitral valve (arrow in Figure A46.2B) is displaced posteriorly toward the left ventricular posterior wall, and that its opening is limited.

In Figure A46.2C, note that the open aortic valve has only two cusps (opening as a "fish mouth").

TAKE-HOME LESSON:

Not all mitral valve deformities indicate anatomic pathology of the mitral valve. The posteriorly directed aortic regurgitation may cause the mitral valve to flutter in diastole, and it may cause a diastolic rumble mimicking mitral stenosis (Austin Flint murmur).

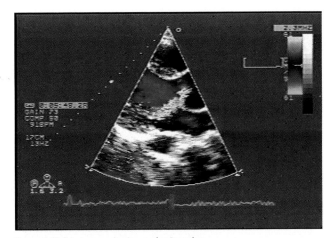

Figure A46.2A: Long-axis view, color Doppler.

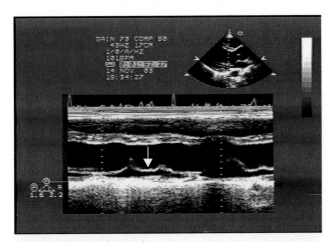

Figure A46.2B: M-mode echo, long axis.

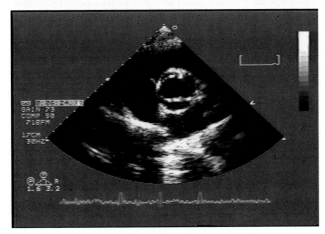

Figure A46.2C: Short-axis view of the aortic valve in systole.

CASE 47 Unique Doppler Pattern

*E*chocardiography was done to evaluate left ventricular obstruction (Figures Q47.1A and Q47.1B). There was normal left ventricular size and wall thickness, with a very high ejection fraction. There was no valvular pathology.

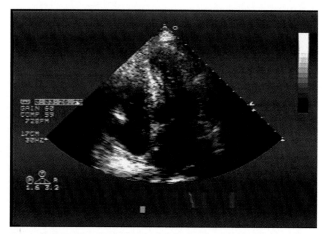

Figure Q47.1A: Two-dimensional echo, apical four-chamber view.

QUESTION 47.1. What does the 3.5-m/second flow (asterisk in Figure Q47.1B) represent?

1. Left ventricular outflow obstruction
2. Early diastolic mitral inflow (E wave)
3. Severe aortic insufficiency
4. Something else

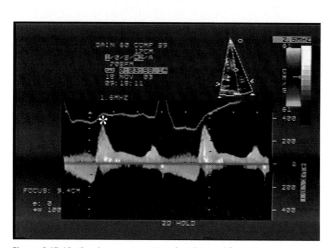

Figure Q47.1B: Continuous wave Doppler obtained from the apex.

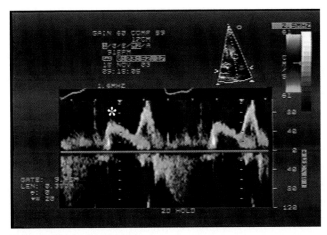

Figure A47.1A: Pulsed Doppler.

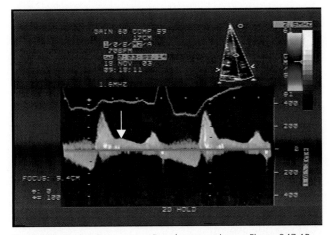

Figure A47.1B: Continuous wave Doppler, same view as Figure Q47.1B.

ANSWER 47.1. Correct answer: 4, something else.

This early diastolic flow is not the E wave of mitral inflow. It is high velocity, representing a gradient of approximately 50 mm Hg, and as noted, there was no valvular pathology. A pulsed Doppler tracing of the mitral inflow is seen in Figure A47.1A.

Note that the E wave of early diastolic transmitral flow (asterisk) is low velocity (60 cm/second) and therefore the 3.5-m/second wave seen on the continuous wave Doppler in Figure Q47.1 B is not the same thing.

In this patient with a very high ejection fraction, there is midleft ventricular cavity obliteration. Blood is trapped in the basal part of the left ventricle when the aortic valve closes. Before mitral opening (during isovolumic relaxation) this same blood moves toward the left ventricular apex as the midcavity obliteration relaxes. It moves with a high velocity because the trapped blood is under higher pressure than the blood at the apex of the left ventricle. The E wave of early diastolic inflow (which occurs when the mitral valve opens, after isovolumic relaxation; arrow), is seen in Figure A47.1B (same continuous wave Doppler view as in Figure Q47.1B).

The arrow points to the low-velocity mitral E wave.

48 More Than Meets the Eye

A 73-year-old man is admitted because of a cerebral embolic event, and is found to be in atrial fibrillation. Transesophageal echocardiography (TEE) is performed. Note the 0.5-mm, round, mobile mass (arrow in Figure Q48.1). There was also some spontaneous echo contrast (smoke) seen.

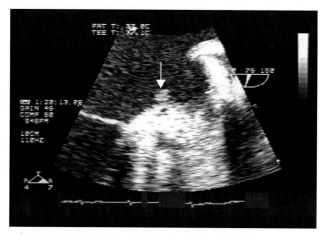

Figure Q48.1: TEE, showing the left atrial appendage.

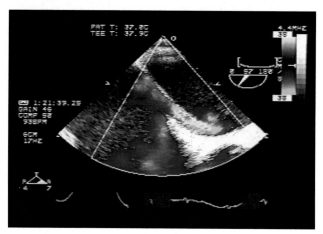

Figure Q48.2: TEE of the midatrial septum.

QUESTION 48.1. What is this mass?

1. Papillary fibroelastoma
2. Myxoma
3. Pectinate muscle (normal finding)
4. Clot

QUESTION 48.2. What would you do?

1. Watchful waiting
2. Prescribe aspirin
3. Prescribe heparin, then warfarin
4. Prescribe plavix
5. Finish the TEE
6. 2 and 4
7. 3 and 5

QUESTION 48.3. The TEE finding in Figure Q48.2 and Figure Q48.3 represents which of the following?

1. Atrial septal defect (ASD)
2. Patent foramen ovale (PFO)
3. Ventricular septal defect (VSD)
4. Tricuspid insufficiency

QUESTION 48.4. That's not all. With the probe withdrawn slightly more superiorly, the following image was obtained (Figure Q48.4). What other abnormality does this patient have?

1. Sinus venosus ASD
2. Primum ASD
3. Secundum ASD
4. Coronary sinus ASD

QUESTION 48.5. Although that is enough for one patient (a left atrial clot, a PFO, and a sinus venosus ASD), finishing the TEE revealed large atherosclerotic plaques in the aortic arch (arrows in Q48.5), with superimposed mobile thrombi (yet another possible source of embolus).

Which one of these was the cause of the cerebral event?

1. Left atrial (LA) clot
2. PFO
3. ASD
4. Aortic plaque
5. No way to tell

ANSWER 48.1. Correct answer: 4, clot. In a patient with atrial fibrillation and spontaneous echo contrast in the left atrium, a mobile mass in or near the left atrial appendage is almost certainly a clot.

ANSWER 48.2. Correct answer: 7, both 3 and 5 are correct. In a 73-year-old patient with atrial fibrillation, a cerebral embolus, and a probable left atrial clot on TEE, anticoagulation with heparin, then warfarin, is the correct therapy. However, barring complications, the TEE should be finished even though the putative diagnosis is established.

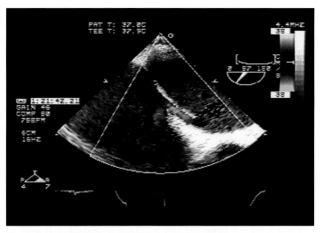

Figure Q48.3: TEE of the midatrial septum, inspiration.

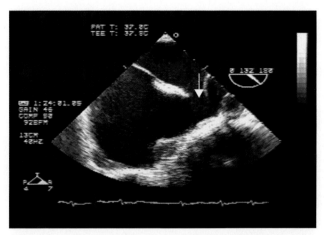

Figure Q48.4: TEE of the superior portion of the atrial septum.

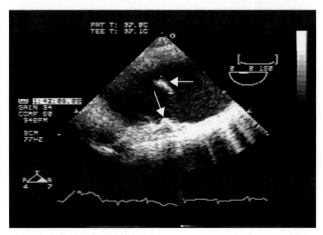

Figure Q48.5: TEE of the aortic arch.

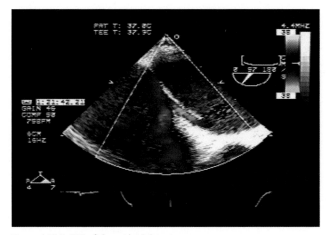

Figure A48.2: TEE of the midatrial septum.

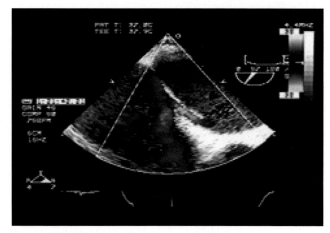

Figure A48.3: TEE of the midatrial septum, inspiration.

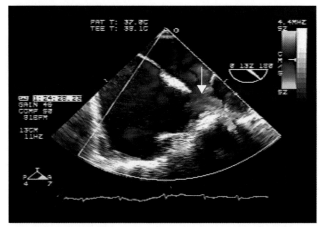

Figure A48.4A: TEE showing the sinus venosus ASD with right-to-left shunting seen in red (arrow).

ANSWER 48.3. Correct answer: 2, PFO. There is a separation between the thinner septum primum and the thicker septum secundum, with blood flow shunting from right to left seen in blue, aliasing to yellow in the center. Figure A48.2 and Figure A48.3 show that blood also shunts from left to right, in red (toward the transducer).

ANSWER 48.4. Correct answer: 1, sinus venosus ASD. There is a defect in the superior part of the atrial septum, representing a sinus venosus ASD. Both pulsed and color Doppler show that there is bidirectional shunting across the ASD, as well as across the PFO, seen previously (Figures A48.4A and A48.4B).

Note that blood flow occurs in both directions-toward the left atrium, above the baseline (right to left) and toward the right atrium, below the baseline (left to right).

ANSWER 48.5. Correct answer: 5, no way to tell. Each of these may be responsible for an embolic event.

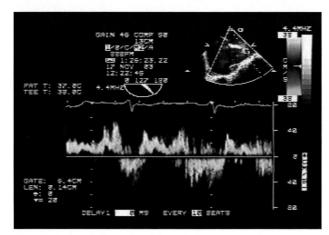

Figure A48.4B: Pulsed Doppler of the ASD shunt.

TAKE-HOME LESSON:
Always do a complete study; you never know what findings will emerge. Although warfarin is indicated to prevent further clot formation in the left atrium, a statin drug is also indicated to prevent plaque instability (and clot embolization) in the aortic arch.

49 Name This Mass

A 56-year-old man was referred for a stress echo because of atypical chest pain. He was referred for a transesophageal echocardiogram (TEE) (Figures Q49.1A through Q49.1C) after transthoracic echocardiography (TTE) suggested a left atrial mass (the stress echo was not performed). He is in normal sinus rhythm and has no previous cardiac history.

The remainder of the TEE examination was normal.

QUESTION 49.1. What is the most likely diagnosis?

1. Myxoma
2. Normal variant
3. Cor triatriatum
4. Clot

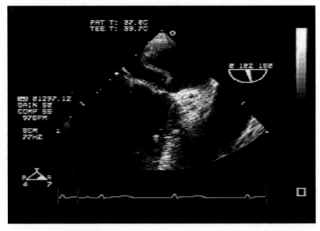

Figure Q49.1B: TEE, same view as Figure Q49.1A, a few frames later in time.

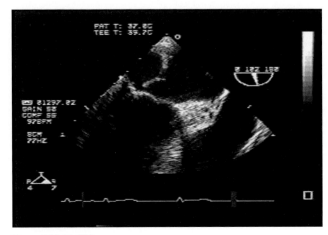

Figure Q49.1A: TEE.

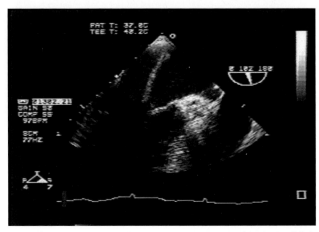

Figure Q49.1C: TEE, same view as Figures Q49.1A and Q49.1B, slightly thereafter.

ANSWER 49.1. Correct answer: 1, myxoma. Although the findings are not typical of myxoma (the mass is not attached to the atrial septum, and it is almost linear and highly mobile), pathologic examination revealed that it was in fact a myxoma. A left atrial clot would be unlikely in a patient with normal sinus rhythm and no spontaneous echo contrast. This patient's coagulation profile was not abnormal. The membrane of cor triatriatum, which divided the left atrium into a proximal and a distal chamber, is not highly mobile and is usually parallel to the left ventricular inflow (mitral valve annulus). We are not aware of any normal variants that present as an elongated, mobile mass in the left atrium.

TAKE-HOME LESSON:

Not all myxomas have a typical appearance.

50 The History Is Key

A 55-year-old man presented with aphasia lasting several minutes. Physical examination was positive only for mild hypertension. His surgical history was positive for removal of a left atrial myxoma 6 years previously. M-mode echo is shown in Figure Q50.1.

QUESTION 50.1. What is the diagnosis?

1. Left atrial myxoma
2. Left ventricular myxoma
3. Mitral valve vegetation
4. Mitral stenosis

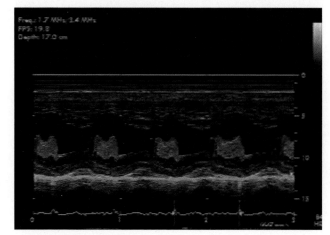

Figure Q50.1: M-mode echo.

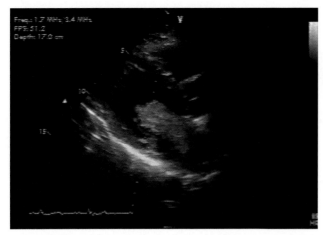

Figure A50.1A: Two-dimensional echo, long-axis view.

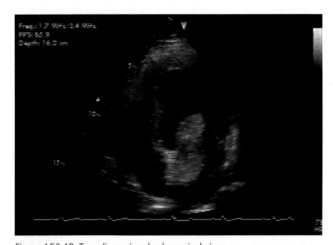

Figure A50.1B: Two-dimensional echo, apical view.

ANSWER 50.1. Correct answer: 1, left atrial myxoma. There is a mass that fills the mitral orifice in diastole, which does not appear in the mitral orifice for a very brief period after the mitral valve opens (note the diagnostic narrow, clear space between the anterior mitral leaflet at the beginning of diastole). This is therefore a left atrial mass that prolapses through the mitral orifice in diastole. In a patient with a previous myxoma, this is almost certainly a recurrent myxoma. This is confirmed on two-dimensional echo in the Figures A50.1A and A50.1B.

TAKE-HOME LESSON:

A rim of normal atrial septum should be resected along with the tumor, to avoid recurrent myxomas.

51 Transesophageal Echocardiograpy (TEE) During Procedure

*T*he pulsed Doppler seen in Figure Q51.1 was obtained before (panel A) and after (panel B) a certain procedure.

QUESTION 51.1. What was the location of the sample volume for this pulsed Doppler?

1. The tip of the mitral leaflets
2. Main pulmonary artery
3. Right upper pulmonary vein
4. Proximal descending aorta
5. Left main coronary artery

QUESTION 51.2. What was the procedure?

1. Balloon mitral valvuloplasty
2. Ablation for atrial fibrillation (AF)
3. Atrial septal defect (ASD) closure
4. Balloon treatment of coarctation of the aorta

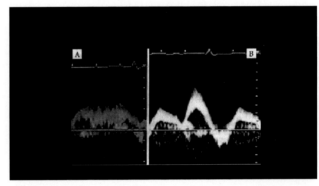

Figure Q51.1: TEE, pulsed Doppler. The scale is 20 cm/second between two vertical points.

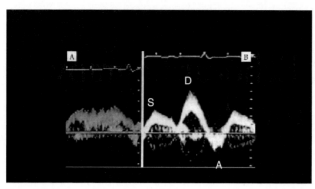

Figure A51.1: Same view as Figure Q51.1.

ANSWER 51.1. Correct answer: 3, right upper pulmonary vein. There is low-velocity flow toward the transducer in both systole and diastole (best seen in panel B), and therefore this is not transmitral flow (which is only diastolic). The flow in the main pulmonary artery on TEE is only systolic. The flow in the descending aorta has a characteristic arterial flow appearance, and is prominently systolic; usually there is no diastolic antegrade flow. Left main coronary artery flow is biphasic (diastolic and systolic). However there is no reversal of flow, as is seen in this pulsed Doppler. By exclusion, this pulsed Doppler therefore represents pulmonary vein flow. The characteristic systolic (S), diastolic (D) and A-reversal (A) flow can be seen in Figure A51.1, panel B.

ANSWER 51.2. Correct answer: 3, ASD closure. Panel A of Figure A51.1 shows typical flow in the pulmonary vein of a patient with a large, uncomplicated ASD with left-to-right shunting. Because most of the blood leaves the left atrium through the ASD (rather than through the mitral valve), the flow characteristics are influenced mainly by the resistance of the ASD rather than that of the left ventricle. The flow in the pulmonary vein will mimic the flow through the ASD, and will occur with similar velocity in systole and diastole (as in Panel A) without obvious separate systolic and diastolic waves. After ASD closure, the flow in the pulmonary vein returns to normal. There is well-formed systolic wave (S) that is the result of the descent of the mitral ring toward the left ventricular apex, as well as atrial relaxation. The diastolic wave (D) is due to the opening of the mitral valve and the pressure gradient between the left atrium and left ventricle. During atrial contraction there is retrograde flow in the pulmonary vein (Label A).

This is not a mitral balloon valvuloplasty, because the velocities are not higher in panel A and lower in panel B. Also, if this were mitral stenosis, the flow should be only in diastole. Pulmonary vein ablation for AF may lead to pulmonary venous stenosis. This may lead to an increase in velocity, but with a loss of the waveforms after the procedure. Also, if the pressure gradient across the pulmonary vein stenosis is high, there will be no reversal of flow with atrial contraction (Lable A). These are not tracings from a coarctation because the velocity is low prior to the procedure, and there would have been high velocity in systole.

52 Malfunctioning Prosthetic Valve?

*T*his 28-year-old man, with a history of intravenous drug addiction, had tricuspid endocarditis in the past. His tricuspid valve was replaced with a tissue prosthesis 4 years ago. The patient now complains of leg edema and upper abdominal pain, and an echocardiogram was done (Figure Q52.1).

QUESTION 52.1. This study shows:

1. Normal tissue prosthesis
2. Prosthetic valve stenosis
3. Prosthetic valve insufficiency
4. Both 2 and 3 are correct

QUESTION 52.2. The patient's central venous pressure (CVP) was measured by catheter, and it was found to be 30 mm Hg. Based on this, and on the Doppler in Figure Q52.1, the estimated pulmonary artery systolic pressure is which of the following?

1. 100 mm Hg
2. 60 mm Hg
3. 42 mm Hg
4. 26 mm Hg

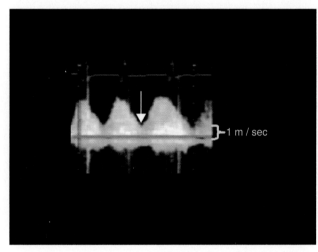

Figure Q52.1: Continuous wave Doppler with the transducer at the apex in an attempt to record tricuspid valve flow.

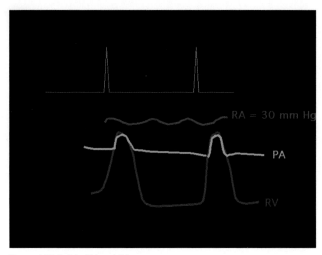

Figure A52.2: RA, RV, and PA pressures.

ANSWER 52.1. Correct answer: 2, prosthetic valve stenosis alone. Note that the antegrade flow across the prosthesis continues throughout the cardiac cycle. This very unusual occurrence is probably the most dramatic finding in very severe tricuspid stenosis. There is a significant gradient across the tricuspid valve not only in diastole (as is usually seen in tricuspid stenosis) but in systole as well. This is because of a huge elevation in right atrial pressure, which is higher than the right ventricular systolic pressure. Obviously, if the right atrial pressure during ventricular systole is higher than the ventricular systolic pressure, tricuspid regurgitation cannot happen.

ANSWER 52.2. Correct answer: 4, 26 mm Hg. This can be calculated from the fact that during ventricular systole, the transtricuspid flow velocity is 1 m/second (arrow, Figure Q52.1), indicating a systolic gradient of 4 mm Hg between the right atrium and right ventricle. Because the CVP (right atrial [RA] pressure) is 30 mm Hg, the right ventricular (RV) systolic pressure (and therefore the pulmonary artery [PA] systolic pressure) is 30 − 4 = 26 mm Hg (Figure A52.2).

Note that the RA pressure is higher than the RV and PA pressures throughout the cardiac cycle.

5.3 Elderly Patient With Syncope

*A*n 81-year-old woman fainted while working in her kitchen. She was brought to the emergency room where her blood pressure measured 110/70 and her pulse was 80 BPM and irregular. The second heard sound was faint, and there was a loud systolic ejection murmur heard at the base with radiation to the neck. An echo was obtained (Figure Q53.1A).

Two-dimensional echo (not shown) showed aortic valve thickening, mild concentric left ventricular hypertrophy, and no systolic anterior motion of the mitral valve or other subaortic obstruction.

An attempt was made to record transaortic valve flow (Figure Q53.1B).

QUESTION 53.1. Based on these findings, what would be your next step?

1. Cardiac catheterization for more hemodynamic data
2. Coronary arteriography followed by aortic valve replacement
3. Aortic valve replacement without coronary arteriography
4. Amyl nitrite inhalation with Doppler measurements
5. Another test

ANSWER 53.1. Correct answer: 5, another test (this is always the right answer, but you have to suggest which one!)

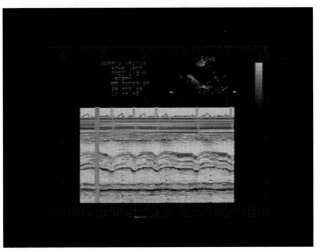

Figure Q53.1A: M-mode of the aortic root, aortic valve, and left atrium.

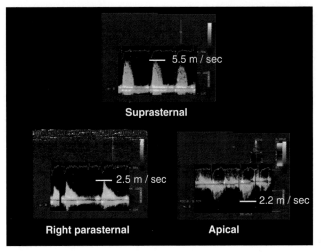

Figure Q53.1B: Doppler echocardiogram.

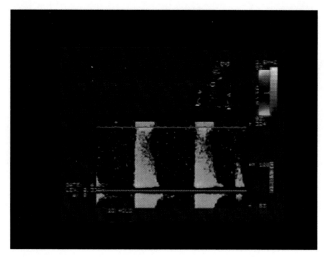

Figure A53.2A: Pulsed Doppler of the right subclavian artery.

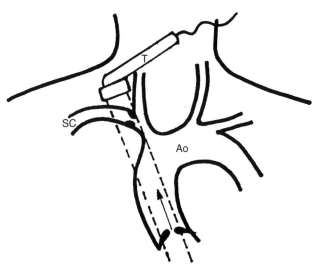

Figure A53.2B: Ao = Aorta; T = Transducer; Dotted line = Ultrasound beam; SC = Subclavian artery. After Otto CM, Miyake-Hull CY, Gardner-CJ, et al. Subclavian artery stenosis masquerading as prosthetic aortic stenosis. *J Am Soc Echo* 1992;5:459–62.

QUESTION 53.2. Which other test would you do?

1. Cardiac magnetic resonance imaging
2. Holter monitoring
3. Tilt table
4. Peripheral vascular Doppler
5. Four-hour glucose tolerance test

ANSWER 53.2. Correct answer: 4, peripheral vascular Doppler. The usual teaching is to select the highest measured Doppler velocity for calculation of the aortic valve gradient. Typically, the fastest velocity reflects the best Doppler angle, that closest to 0 degrees. In this patient not only is the velocity lower from two windows, but the shape of the parasternal and apical flow velocity spectral tracings is also quite different. The shape shows early peaking, indicating a lack of severe stenosis. The late-peaking high-velocity flow recorded from suprasternal window is altogether different. The M-mode echo in Figure Q53.1A shows that the aortic valve, although thickened, has a fairly good excursion. This finding is unlikely in an elderly patient if the aortic valve velocity were really 5.5 m/second (a gradient of 121 mm Hg). Based on all of this, it was assumed that the late-peaking high velocity recorded from the parasternal window was due to something else. In fact, Doppler interrogation of the subclavian artery showed severe proximal narrowing in this vessel (Figure A53.2A).

The sample volume is just distal to a high-grade stenosis at the origin of the right subclavian artery. Note flow velocity aliasing at nearly 4 m/second.

It should always be kept in mind that continuous wave Doppler has no depth resolution. Figure A53.2B shows how subclavian stenosis can give the false impression of aortic stenosis. On further interrogation, our patient told us that she fainted after she was trying to reach something on top of her refrigerator. It is therefore probable that exercising her right arm produced a subclavian steal syndrome. A more detailed physical examination showed a discrepancy in the blood pressures of the left and right arms (there was a 100-mm Hg difference).

TAKE-HOME LESSON:

A thorough physical examination may be more informative than more sophisticated, expensive tests.

54 Chest Pain in a Patient With Aortic Plaque

*T*his 75-year-old patient was admitted to the hospital with severe chest pain. Three weeks previously he had a short episode of aphasia and right-arm numbness. This transesophageal echocardiogram (TEE) was done prior to coronary angiography (Figure Q54.1). There was only mild atherosclerosis of the ascending aorta.

QUESTION 54.1. What would you recommend to the interventional cardiologist?

1. Ignore the finding
2. Cancel the procedure, it's too risky
3. Give anticoagulation for 3 weeks, then repeat the TEE
4. Do the angiogram from the right brachial artery

QUESTION 54.2. How would you instruct the surgeon?

1. Abort the operation, it's too risky
2. Proceed with open heart surgery because the patient is at risk
3. Perform aortic arch endarterectomy, and then coronary bypass
4. Perform off-pump coronary artery bypass

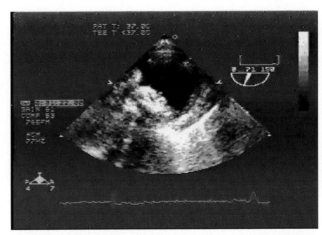

Figure Q54.1: TEE of the aortic arch.

QUESTION 54.3. The patient survived the surgery and is about to be discharged from the hospital. The only drug that has been shown to prevent embolization in patients with severe aortic plaque on TEE (in a retrospective study [Tunick, et al]) is a statin. In addition to a statin, what would you recommend?

1. Aspirin
2. Warfarin
3. Plavix
4. I'm not sure

ANSWER 54.1. Correct answer: 4, do the coronary angiogram from the right brachial artery. By doing that, you are less likely to negotiate the atheroma-laden mid and distal aortic arch (most likely the descending aorta will also have severe plaque, which will be avoided).

Coronary angiography revealed severe triple vessel disease not amenable to angioplasty. In spite of medical therapy, the patient continues to have angina, and surgery is recommended.

ANSWER 54.2. This patient is too sick to abort the procedure. Cannulation of the aortic arch in patients with severe arch plaque is very high risk (intraoperative stroke rate = 12%). Aortic endarterectomy has an even higher risk (34%). Therefore the correct answer is 4, off-pump coronary artery bypass. Without aortic manipulation, the risk of stroke decreases significantly.

ANSWER 54.3. Correct answer: 4, I'm not sure. Retrospective data show a benefit of statins, but no difference between antiplatelet drugs and warfarin in preventing embolization in patients with severe aortic plaque on TEE. Until the results are available from a prospective multicenter randomized trial of warfarin and antiplatelet drugs, there are no good data pointing to one or the other.

55 Syncope and Murmur

A 63-year-old woman fainted. A systolic murmur was heard at the base, radiating to the carotids. On two-dimensional echo the aortic valve was thickened and partially calcified. There was no left ventricular outflow obstruction. There was mild left ventricular hypertrophy (LVH) and a normal ejection fraction. A continuous wave Doppler was obtained (Figure Q55.1).

QUESTION 55.1. Based on the clinical history and this Doppler finding, what would you recommend?

1. Left- and right-heart catheterization and coronary angiography
2. Aortic valve replacement after coronary angiography
3. Dobutamine stress echo
4. Transesophageal echocardiography (TEE)
5. None of the above

QUESTION 55.2. The patient's attending physician decided to refer the patient for cardiac catheterization. It showed that the mean aortic valve gradient was only 10 mm Hg, and the aortic valve area was 1.6 cm^2 (there was only mild aortic stenosis [AS] on catheterization). Because of the cath results, the echo was reviewed, and an additional continuous wave Doppler spectral tracing was found (Figure Q55.2). Who messed up?

1. We did (the echo lab)
2. They did (the cath lab)
3. He did (the patient)
4. The usual suspects (the insurance company)

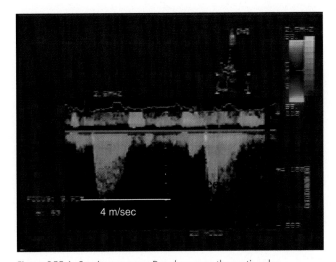

Figure Q55.1: Continuous wave Doppler across the aortic valve.

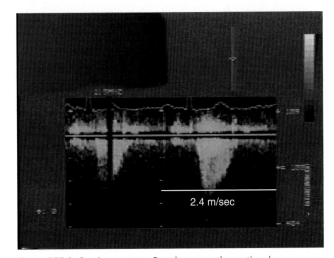

Figure Q55.2: Continuous wave Doppler across the aortic valve.

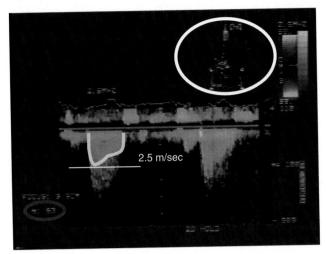

Figure A55.2A: Same view as Figure Q55.1.

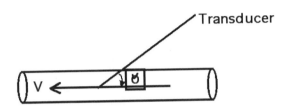

$$\text{Corrected (true) } V = \frac{\text{Observed } V}{\text{Cos } \theta}$$

(Cos θ is always ≤ 1)

Figure A55.2B: Angle correction.

ANSWER 55.1. Correct answer: 5, none of the above. For an explanation, please read on.

ANSWER 55.2. Correct answer: 1, we did (the echo lab). It is difficult to admit, but the first Doppler was incorrectly done. In addition to the difference in peak velocity, there are several differences between Figures Q55.1 and Q55.2. The two Dopplers were performed using different transducers. Figure Q55.1 was performed with an imaging transducer (white oval in Figure A55.2A).

Figure Q55.2 was performed using a stand-alone non-imaging continuous wave (CW) transducer. If you pay close attention you will see a second, lower velocity buried in the spectral tracing in Figure Q55.1 (the yellow line in Figure A55.2A). This denser (whiter) tracing represents the left ventricular outflow velocity, which reaches a velocity of 2.5 m/second. The ratio between the transvalvular velocity and the outflow tract velocity on this tracing is only 1.6, which indicates that the aortic stenosis can only be mild. The ratio should be 4 or more in severe aortic stenosis. It is interesting that the same exact ratio (1.6) is present also in Figure Q55.2. How then to explain the discrepancy? The answer lies in Figure A55.2B.

The angle correction feature is present on the imaging transducer but not on the nonimaging CW transducer. When blood flow is not parallel to the direction of the ultrasound beam, angle correction may be used in order to correct for the fact that there is too great an angle of incidence between the ultrasound beam and the direction of flow. In this case, the angle correction was incorrectly set too high, yielding a falsely high velocity. In fact, the angle correction used appears (red circle on Figure Q55.2). It shows that the angle correction was 63 degrees (although this is not distinctly visible in our figure). Figure Q55.2, without angle correction, is therefore the true transaortic valve velocity, and this patient indeed has only mild AS.

TAKE-HOME LESSON:

Echo machines are complicated, and great care must be taken to prevent artifacts. In this case an unnecessary cardiac catheterization was done, but luckily no one sent the patient for aortic valve replacement.

56 Enlarged Heart

Cardiomegaly was found in this 57-year-old asymptomatic woman. The physical examination revealed a systolic murmur at the left sternal border, and therefore an echocardiogram was ordered. The transthoracic echocardiogram (TTE) showed a dilated right ventricle and no evidence of significant tricuspid or pulmonic regurgitation or intracardiac shunt. Transesophageal echocardiography (TEE) was done (Figures Q56.1A through Q56.1C).

QUESTION 56.1. What are these studies suggestive of?

1. Atrial septal defect (ASD)
2. Left-to-right shunt
3. Right-to-left shunt
4. Tricuspid atresia

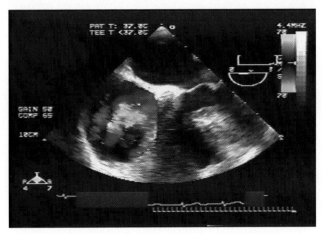

Figure Q56.1B: Same view as Q56.1A, with color Doppler.

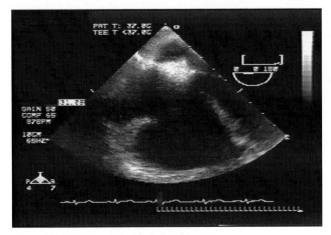

Figure Q56.1A: TEE, modified four-chamber view.

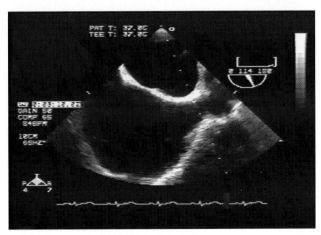

Figure Q56.1C: TEE, bicaval view of right atrium.

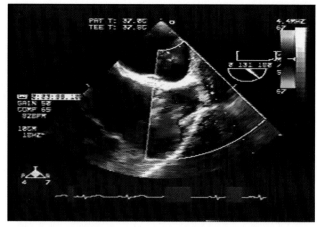

Figure Q56.2: Same view as Figure Q56.1C, with color Doppler.

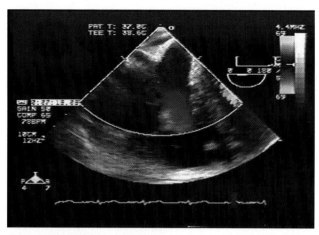

Figure Q56.3: TEE of the right atrium.

QUESTION 56.2. What is the cause of the dilated right atrium and right ventricle seen in Figure Q56.2?

1. Tricuspid insufficiency
2. Pulmonary embolus
3. Anomalous pulmonary vein
4. Arrhythmogenic right ventricular dysplasia

QUESTION 56.3. What is the associated anomaly in Figure Q56.3?

1. Persistent left superior vena cava
2. Patent ductus arteriosus
3. Noncompaction of the right ventricle
4. Rhabdomyoma

ANSWER 56.1. Correct answer: 2, left-to-right shunt. There is a dilated right atrium and right ventricle (Figure Q56.1A). Although there is more color flow seen in the right atrium than in the left atrium (Figure Q56.1B), there is no defect seen in the atrial septum (Figure Q56.1C). Patients with a right-to-left shunt and dilated heart chambers are cyanotic or otherwise symptomatic. Tricuspid atresia would not cause an enlarged right ventricle (just the opposite).

Therefore, there must be something else causing a dilated right heart, such as a left-to-right shunt.

ANSWER 56.2. Correct answer: 3, anomalous pulmonary vein. There is an abnormal flow entering the superior vena cava. Flow is toward the transducer (seen in red, Figure Q56.2). This anomalous vein resulted in a 1.7:1 left-to-right shunt, and therefore the right heart dilatation. It is unusual that the atrial septum is intact (no sinus venosus ASD). However, there is another anomaly present.

ANSWER 56.3. Correct answer: 1, persistent left superior vena cava. Figure Q56.3 shows a dilated coronary sinus entering the right atrium (note the color flow in the coronary sinus [CS] and right atrium [RA], in blue). The coronary sinus is dilated because there is a persistent left superior vena cava entering it (not shown, but confirmed by agitated saline injection into the left arm, which appeared in the dilated CS). This venous abnormality is more common in patients with a sinus venosus ASD (which our patient did not have). However it may also be associated with anomalous pulmonary venous return.

CASE 57 What Is the Left Ventricular Pressure?

A continuous wave Doppler was obtained from a patient with significant aortic stenosis and regurgitation (Figure Q57.1). The blood pressure was 150/80 mm Hg.

Note that both the peak transaortic velocity and the end-diastolic aortic regurgitation velocity are 4 m/second.

QUESTION 57.1. What is the best estimate of left ventricular (LV) pressure?

1. 95/16
2. 214/16
3. 214/44
4. 195/16

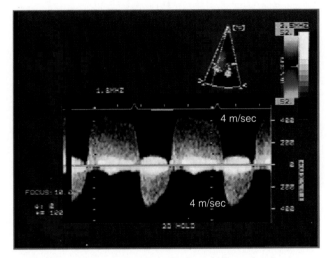

Figure Q57.1: Continuous wave Doppler through the aortic valve.

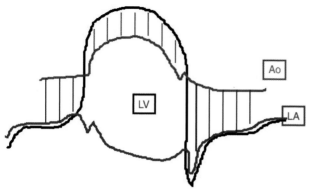

Figure A57.1A: The tracings represent the aortic, left ventricular, and left atrial pressures.

1. Peak - to - Peak Gradient (PP)
2. Maximum Instantaneous Gradient (MIG)
3. Mean Gradient

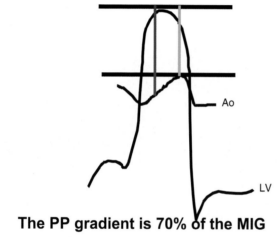

The PP gradient is 70% of the MIG

Figure A57.1B: Aortic gradient.

ANSWER 57.1. The correct answer is 4, 195/16.

We assume that the systolic aortic pressure equals the systolic blood pressure. By adding the transaortic valve gradient to the aortic systolic pressure, one can calculate the left ventricular systolic pressure (Figure A57.1A). Also, by subtracting the aortic regurgitant gradient at end-diastole, one can define the left ventricular end-diastolic pressure. If all of this is true, why is answer 2 incorrect?

The peak aortic gradient measured by Doppler is the maximum instantaneous gradient (Figure A57.1B). This is always higher than the peak-to-peak gradient, which is about 70% of the maximum instantaneous gradient. In order to calculate LV systolic pressure, we are interested in the gradient between the peak LV systolic pressure and the peak aortic pressure. Therefore, although the echo gives us the maximum instantaneous gradient, we have to multiply this by 70% to get the left ventricular peak systolic pressure. The LV pressure is therefore the aortic systolic pressure (150) plus 70% of the maximum instantaneous gradient (64). It is therefore 150 + 45 = 195 mm Hg. Interestingly, this problem does not exist with the diastolic pressure. Therefore, the LV diastolic pressure is 80 – 64 = 16 mm Hg.

58 Elderly Patient With Abdominal Pain

*A*n 85-year-old woman presented with cramping abdominal pain. Workup revealed an elevated amylase and guaiac positive stool. Because of renal insufficiency, a contrast computed tomography scan was not performed, and a transesophageal echocardiogram (TEE) was ordered. A mass was found (Figure Q58.1), and the heart was otherwise normal.

QUESTION 58.1. What would you do?

1. Start the patient on intravenous (IV) heparin.
2. Start the patient on oral warfarin
3. Schedule surgery for the left atrial myxoma
4. Schedule surgery for the right atrial myxoma
5. Finish the TEE

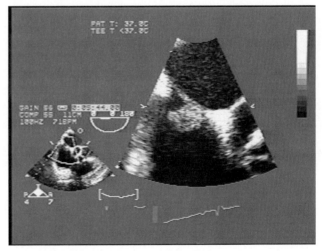

Figure Q58.1: TEE at 0 degrees showing both atria.

QUESTION 58.2. Figure Q58.2 is the finished TEE. What would you do now?

1. Start the patient on IV heparin
2. Start the patient on oral warfarin
3. Start the patient on a statin
4. Schedule surgery for the left atrial myxoma
5. Schedule surgery for the right atrial myxoma

ANSWER 58.1. Correct answer: 5, Finish the TEE. This is always the right answer!

ANSWER 58.2. Correct answer: 3, Start the patient on a statin. Figure Q58.1 shows a right (not a left) atrial myxoma. This is not the cause of the patient's abdominal pain, high amylase, guaiac positive stool, and renal insufficiency. Because the heart was otherwise normal (no patent foramen ovale) there have been no paradoxical emboli. The severe atherosclerotic plaque in the descending aorta seen in Figure Q58.2 is the likely cause of emboli, which are responsible for the clinical picture. Because statins have been shown to be associated with a significant reduction in the frequency of such emboli (in a large, retrospective study [Tunick, et al]), this is the right treatment. Anticoagulation with heparin and/or warfarin has been shown to be inferior to statins for the prevention of emboli from aortic plaque, and the patient is having gastrointestinal bleeding, making these drugs relatively contraindicated. Removal of an asymptomatic right atrial myxoma in an 85-year-old patient with renal failure and intestinal infarction (bleeding) is too hazardous at the present time.

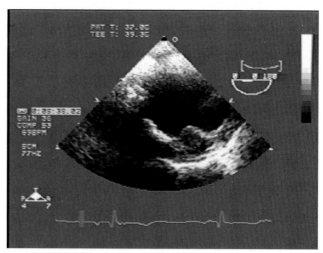

Figure Q58.2: TEE of the descending thoracic aorta.

TAKE-HOME LESSON:

Always do a complete echocardiographic examination, even when you think the diagnosis may be already established.

59 Edema

A 46-year-old woman was admitted with the recent onset of bilateral edema to both knees and fatigue. She had a history of a St. Jude's aortic valve replacement (bileaflet tilting disk valve) 2 years previously. She was afebrile. The INR was 1.8. Because of the recent symptoms, a transesophageal echocardiogram (TEE) was done (Figures Q59.1A and Q59.1B). There was no valvular stenosis or regurgitation, and the pulmonary artery pressure was normal.

QUESTION 59.1. Based on these images, what is the cause of the patient's symptoms?

1. Myocardial infarction
2. Inferior vena cava syndrome
3. Cardiac tamponade
4. Myocardial abscess
5. Pulmonary embolus

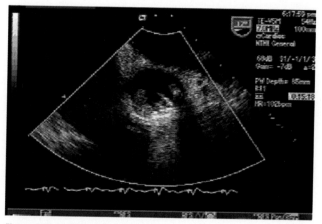

Figure Q59.1A: TEE of the aortic root.

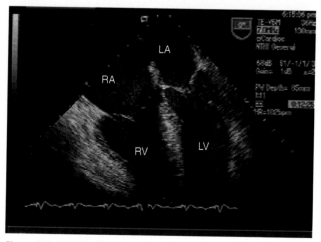

Figure Q59.1B: TEE of both ventricles; Left ventricle function was normal but the RV was hypokinetic.

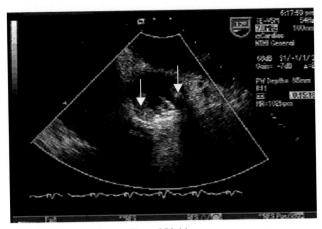

Figure A59.1: Same view as Figure Q59.1A.

ANSWER 59.1. Correct answer: 1, myocardial infarction. This one is tough. Figure Q59.1A shows that there is thrombus around the leaflets of the aortic prosthesis (see arrows, Figure A59.1). While vegetations may have a similar appearance, the patient's history is not suggestive of endocarditis. On the other hand, her INR was subtherapeutic, especially for a mechanical prosthesis. The thrombus is in the region of the right coronary ostium, around the anterior aspect of the aorta. The four-chamber view in Figure Q59.1B shows that the right atrium (RA) and right ventricle (RV) are both dilated. In the absence of tricuspid valve disease and pulmonary hypertension, right ventricular infarction is the most likely option. Indeed, the RV was severely hypokinetic.

Inferior vena cava syndrome will not cause a dilated right heart. There is also no evidence of pericardial effusion, and both the history and the images are not suggestive of endocarditis (myocardial abscess). It is unlikely to be a pulmonary embolus because the pulmonary artery (PA) pressure is normal; therefore pulmonary embolus is unlikely to be the cause of RV hypokinesis.

TAKE-HOME LESSON:
Coronary artery embolization should always be considered in an unstable patient with a prosthetic valve.

60 Elderly Woman With Chronic Obstructive Pulmonary Disease

*T*his 75-year-old woman has been treated for chronic obstructive pulmonary disease (COPD). An echocardiogram was ordered because of mild dyspnea on exertion and an abnormal chest x-ray. She had only mild tricuspid regurgitation, with a normal velocity (no evidence of pulmonary hypertension).

The pulsed Doppler of the flow toward the transducer (red flow) seen in Figure Q60.1A is shown in Figure Q60.1B

QUESTION 60.1. What syndrome does this patient have?

1. Budd-Chiari syndrome
2. Hepatopulmonary syndrome (portopulmonary hypertension)
3. Malignant inferior vena cava (IVC) syndrome
4. Scimitar syndrome

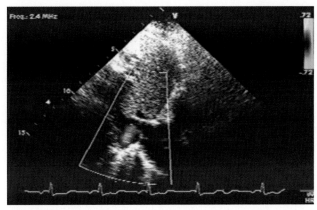

Figure Q60.1A: Subxiphoid view.

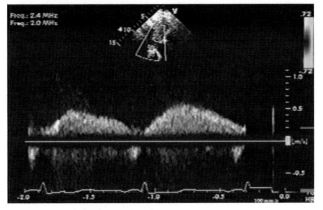

Figure Q60.1B: Pulsed wave Doppler.

ANSWER 60.1. Correct answer: 4, Scimitar syndrome. The red flow seen in Figure Q60.1A enters the IVC just proximal to the right atrium. This is flow from an anomalous pulmonary vein draining into the IVC. The patient has atresia of the right middle and right upper pulmonary lobes, along with an anomalous arterial supply to her right lung from the abdominal aorta and the anomalous pulmonary vein seen here. There is a second, smaller right-sided pulmonary vein that takes a circuitous course but eventually drains normally into the left atrium (seen on computed tomography). Her heart is slightly dextroposed (because of the right lung atresia). This is called Scimitar syndrome because of the characteristic curved shadow to the right of the heart on chest x-ray (shaped like a Turkish sword, or scimitar), which is due to the anomalous veins. In some cases, the anomalous veins drain into the portal system rather than the IVC. When the shunt is large, surgical correction is required in the neonatal period. This patient has only one anomalous vein, and her right atrium and right ventricle are not enlarged. Her pulmonary artery pressure is normal. Therefore, she remains relatively asymptomatic, and no surgical correction is indicated.

Answers 1 and 3 are not correct because there is no evidence of obstruction of the hepatic veins or the IVC. Answer 2 is incorrect because of the normal tricuspid regurgitation velocity (normal pulmonary artery pressure).

61 Murmur

*T*his 45-year-old woman has a heart murmur detected on a routine physical examination. She is asymptomatic. An echocardiogram is ordered (Figure Q61.1).

QUESTION 61.1. Which of the following is (are) true?

1. The mitral regurgitation (MR) is going clockwise (down the lateral wall of the left atrium, and up the interatrial septum)
2. The MR is going counter-clockwise (down the interatrial septum and up the lateral wall of the left atrium)
3. The patient has anterior leaflet mitral prolapse
4. The patient has posterior leaflet mitral prolapse
5. Both 1 and 3 are correct
6. Both 2 and 4 are correct

QUESTION 61.2. Where will the systolic murmur radiate?

1. To the axilla
2. To the base
3. To the back
4. To the neck
5. Both 1 and 3 are correct
6. Both 2 and 4 are correct

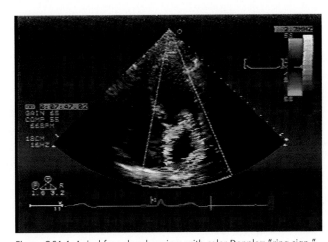

Figure Q61.1: Apical four-chamber view, with color Doppler: "ring sign."

ANSWER 61.1. Correct answer: 6, both 2 and 4 are correct. When the posterior leaflet is prolapsing, the MR is directed anteriorly, under the anterior leaflet and along the interatrial septum. In this example, the MR takes a completely circular path and heads counter-clockwise along the interatrial septum and then up the lateral wall of the left atrium.

ANSWER 61.2. Correct answer: 6, both 2 and 4 are correct. Because the MR is directed anteriorly, it proceeds under the aortic root. Because of this, the murmur radiates to the base of the heart (second left interspace) and to the neck (carotids). It can be distinguished from aortic stenosis because of the brisk carotid upstrokes.

62 Hole in the Right Atrium?

One year after successful mitral valve repair, this patient developed neck vein distention but no leg edema. The echocardiogram showed the mitral annuloplasty ring with only minimal mitral regurgitation (not shown here). The four-chamber and subxiphoid views are shown in Figures Q62.1A through Q62.1D.

QUESTION 62.1. Which finding do these echo images NOT show?

1. Severe tricuspid regurgitation (TR)
2. Dilated right atrium (RA)
3. Rupture of the free wall of the RA with pseudoaneurysm formation
4. Pacing wires for dual chamber pacing

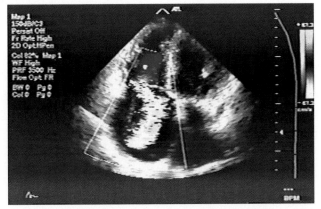

Figure Q62.1B: Same view as Figure Q62.1A, with color Doppler.

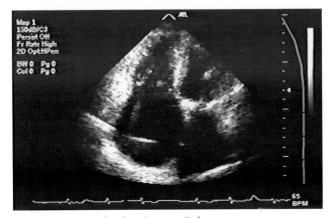

Figure Q62.1A: Four-chamber view, systolic frame.

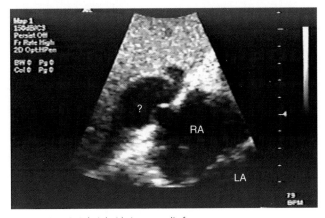

Figure Q62.1C: Subxiphoid view, systolic frame.

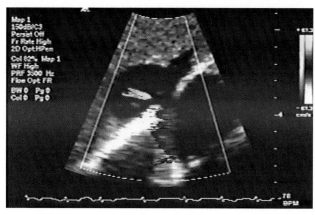

Figure Q62.1D: Same view as Figure Q62.1C, with color Doppler.

QUESTION 62.2. Based on these echo images, how do you explain the fact that the patient has neck vein distention but no leg edema?

1. The RA pressure is not elevated
2. The inferior vena cava (IVC) pressure is not elevated
3. The superior vena cava (SVC) pressure is not elevated
4. Mediastinal fibrosis

ANSWER 62.1. Correct answer: 3, rupture of the free wall of the RA with pseudoaneurysm (this is NOT present). The dilated structure outside the RA is a dilated IVC at its junction with the RA. Tilting the transducer shows more of the IVC, and the rest of the IVC is not dilated (Figure A62.1).

ANSWER 62.2. Correct answer: 2, the IVC pressure is not elevated. This explains the lack of edema. Although SVC syndrome will also cause neck vein distention without leg edema, there is nothing on these images to suggest this or mediastinal fibrosis.

Figure A62.2A shows a eustachian valve (arrow) bulging into the IVC during systole, when the RA pressure is markedly elevated because of the severe TR (seen in Figure Q62.1B). The eustachian valve is a normal structure between the IVC and the RA, which directs blood from the lower half of the body toward the foramen ovale in the fetus. Normally this valve is open throughout the cardiac cycle. In our patient this embryonic remnant is obstructing the opening of the IVC into the RA in systole, therefore preventing transmission of the elevated RA pressure to the IVC in systole. There is only slight eustachian valve insufficiency, seen in color in Figure Q62.1D. In diastole, the eustachian valve is open (Figure A62.2B). Although the IVC is very dilated near the RA, it is not dilated in the rest of its course (see Figure A62.1).

TAKE-HOME LESSON:

The other cardiac valves function to let blood flow in only one direction. Usually the eustachian valve does not prevent regurgitation of blood from the RA into the IVC. However, in this unusual case, it does. As a result, the patient has the rare syndrome of neck vein distention without lower extremity edema, despite high RA pressure.

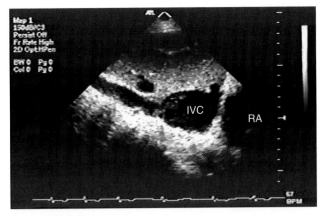

Figure A62.1: IVC.

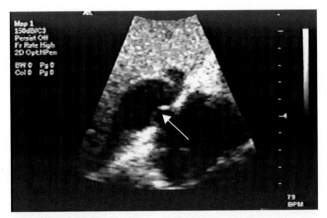

Figure A62.2A: Same view as Figure Q62.1C.

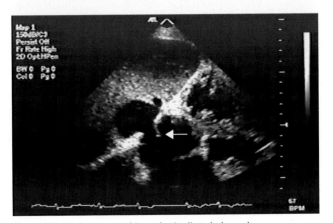

Figure A62.2B: Open eustachian valve in diastole (arrow).

63 Where Is the Infection?

*T*ransesophageal echocardiography (TEE) was performed in a 40-year-old man with endocarditis (Figure Q63.1).

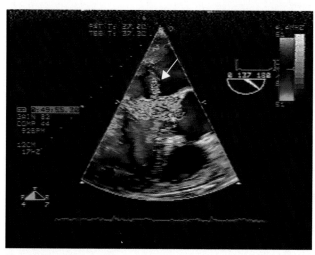

Figure Q63.1: TEE, 137 degrees, diastolic frame.

QUESTION 63.1. Which valve is infected?

1. Aortic
2. Mitral
3. Both
4. Neither

QUESTION 63.2. What is the reason for the color jet of mitral regurgitation (MR) (arrow) in the left atrium (LA) in diastole?

1. This is an artifact related to the relatively low frame rate
2. The color map is set incorrectly
3. The left ventricular (LV) pressure is higher than the left atrial (LA) pressure at this point in diastole
4. There is no MR; the jet (arrow) is from the left atrium into the left ventricle

ANSWER 63.1. Correct answer: 3, both.

ANSWER 63.2. Correct answer: 3, the LV pressure is higher than the LA pressure at this point in diastole.

This patient has aortic insufficiency secondary to aortic valve endocarditis. The jet of aortic regurgitation is impinging on the anterior mitral leaflet, and it created a jet lesion, which is a nidus for further infection on the intact mitral valve. An aneurysm has formed on the anterior mitral leaflet (arrow, Figure A63.1A) and this has perforated, resulting in mitral regurgitation (arrow, Figure A63.1B, showing the more severe systolic regurgitation).

The reason for the diastolic mitral regurgitation seen in Figure Q63.1 may be the result of premature closure of the mitral valve (seen in patients with acute severe aortic regurgitation). The elevation in diastolic LV pressure exceeds the LA pressure in these cases, resulting in regurgitation through the perforation in the closed mitral valve. Another possible mechanism is that the high-velocity diastolic jet of aortic regurgitation hits the anterior mitral leaflet, with some blood crossing into the left atrium across the open mitral valve.

To identify the fact that the mitral regurgitation is indeed through the perforation in the aneurysm of the anterior mitral leaflet, it is useful to freeze a frame and use the "color suppress" feature, as was done in the split-frame views in Figure A63.1B. The flow acceleration and proximal isovelocity surface area (PISA) clearly point to the location of the perforation in the anterior mitral leaflet (Figure A63.2).

> *TAKE-HOME LESSON:*
> **Most perforations in a previously normal anterior mitral leaflet are due to aneurysm formation in the leaflet in patients with aortic regurgitation due to aortic valve endocarditis.**

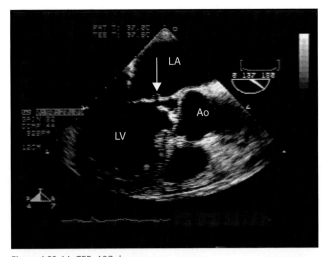

Figure A63.1A: TEE, 137 degrees.

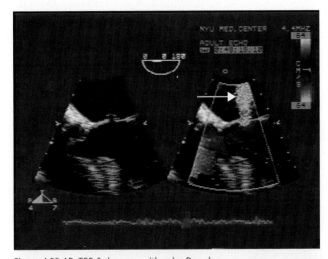

Figure A63.1B: TEE 0 degrees, with color Doppler.

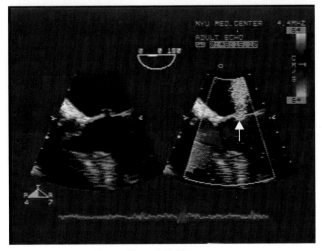

Figure A63.2: Same view as Figure A63.1B.

64 Prosthetic Valve Dysfunction?

A 58-year old woman underwent mitral valve replacement with a Bjork-Shiley tilting disk valve 16 years ago. She was well until recently when she began to complain of dyspnea. On physical examination she was in atrial fibrillation (which was chronic). There were no murmurs. The chest x-ray showed pulmonary congestion. Echocardiography showed normal motion of the prosthetic valve (Figures Q64.1A and Q64.1B).

Transesophageal echocardiography (TEE) did not add any new information: The valve opening appeared to be normal and there was no mitral regurgitation.

A continuous wave Doppler was obtained (Figure Q64.1C). The peak gradient was 21.8 mm Hg, and the mean gradient was 7 mm Hg. The pressure half-time was 100 msec.

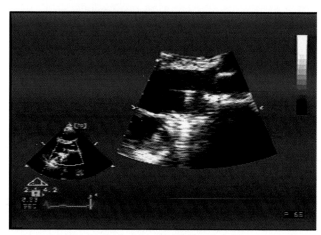

Figure Q64.1A: Transthoracic echo, diastolic frame.

QUESTION 64.1. Based on this information, what would you do?
1. Replace the prosthesis
2. Send the patient to a pulmonologist
3. Send the patient to a psychiatrist
4. Follow-up in 6 months, after changing medical therapy
5. Dobutamine stress echo

QUESTION 64.2. Although this prosthetic valve malfunction is diagnosable from the continuous wave Doppler, it was missed initially and the two-dimensional echo was considered to be normal (both on TEE and transthoracic echocardiography). What is the reason for this?
1. Blood flow was not parallel to the transducer
2. The recording technique was inappropriate
3. The electrocardiogram was not connected correctly
4. The gain settings were incorrect
5. There was a short circuit in the transducer wire

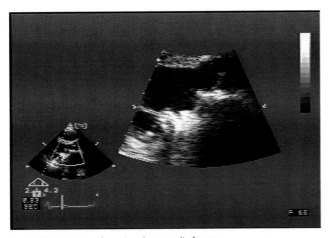

Figure Q64.1B: Transthoracic echo, systolic frame.

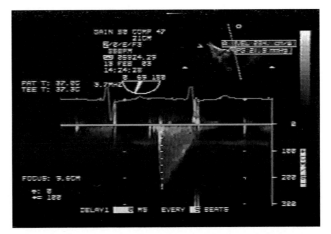

Figure Q64.1C. TEE, continuous wave Doppler of transmitral flow.

ANSWER 64.1. The correct answer is 1, replace the prosthesis. As can be seen from Figure Q64.1C, although three diastolic periods appear on this image, there is diastolic flow across the valve during only one of them. This reflects the fact that the prosthetic valve does not open on every beat. The gradient across the mitral valve was insufficient to open the valve with each beat, and it opened only every other beat. It required two diastolic filling periods of the left atrium for the left atrial pressure to rise to a sufficient degree to open the valve. Once the valve started its opening and the disk escaped the pannus (which was found at surgery), it opened freely, producing a normal appearance and a nearly normal pressure half-time on that cycle. Because the pressure gradient at the onset of valve opening was high, the flow velocity across the valve was also high.

ANSWER 64.2. The correct answer is 2, the recording technique was inappropriate. Many laboratories are utilizing digital storage of echocardiographic images, frequently capturing only a single cardiac cycle per view, which is then played in an endless loop for the interpreting cardiologist to review. Unfortunately, if an abnormality occurs in a cyclical or intermittent fashion, reviewing only a single cardiac cycle may miss it, as was the case with our patient. Figures Q64.1A and Q64.1B are digital images from a single cardiac cycle during which the valve does open.

TAKE-HOME LESSON:

New, more expensive digital equipment is not necessarily more accurate. For certain cases, multiple consecutive cardiac cycles must be digitized. It may be better to use your videotapes if the diagnosis is not clear from the digital loops.

ACKNOWLEDGMENT

Ellis Lader, MD, Mid-Valley Hospital, Kingston, New York.

CASE

65 How Thin Can It Get?

A 48-year-old female presents with hemoptysis and dyspnea. She has a history of paroxysmal supraventricular tachycardia (SVT), and the initial admission electrocardiogram showed nonsustained ventricular tachycardia (VT). Transthoracic echo was suboptimal, and a transesophageal echocardiogram (TEE) was performed (Figures Q65.1A and Q65.1B).

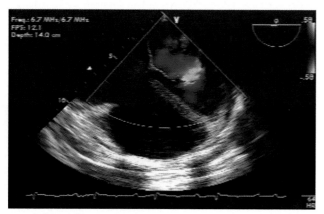

Figure Q65.1A: TEE, four-chamber view.

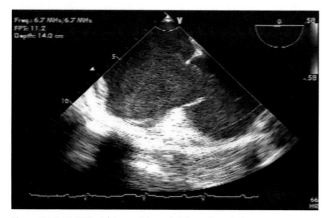

Figure Q65.1B: TEE, right ventricle and right atrium, 0 degrees.

QUESTION 65.1. Why does color flow Doppler show no color on the right side of the heart?

1. The color Doppler was only interrogating the mitral valve
2. Color is usually not seen well farther from the transducer
3. There is something wrong with the patient
4. There is something wrong with the equipment
5. There is something wrong with the insurance company (right-sided color is not reimbursable!)

QUESTION 65.2. What is wrong with the patient?

1. Tricuspid atresia
2. Carcinoid syndrome
3. Behçet's syndrome
4. Uhl's anomaly

QUESTION 65.3. This patient has a central venous pressure catheter that shows that the right atrial (RA) pressure is 20 mm Hg.

What is the pulmonary artery (PA) pressure?

1. 100/40
2. 25/20
3. 25/10
4. 70/30

ANSWER 65.1. The correct answer is 3, there is something wrong with the patient. Note that the color window covers the entire tricuspid orifice and most of the right ventricle and right atrium. Color Doppler signals can be seen at any depth within the color window. This patient has very slow flow within the right heart, as evidenced by the spontaneous echo contrast ("smoke") seen in Figure Q65.1B.

ANSWER 65.2. The correct answer is 4, Uhl's anomaly. In this congenital disorder, right ventricular myocardium is absent. It is replaced by fibro-fatty tissue. This is the most extreme form of right ventricular (RV) dysplasia, and while it usually presents in infancy, some patients survive to adulthood. This patient has an extremely thin-walled right ventricle, approximately 1 to 2 mm. This ventricle does not contract at all, and the tricuspid valve remains open throughout the cardiac cycle (Figure A65.2).

Note the low-velocity flow across the tricuspid valve throughout systole and diastole.

ANSWER 65.3. The correct answer is 2, 25/20. This patient does not have a pumping right ventricle. This can be seen on Figure A65.2 (which hardly shows any phasic flow across the tricuspid valve) and also on Figure A65.3 (which shows low-velocity, almost continuous flow across the pulmonic valve). Without the pumping function of the right ventricle, the whole right side functions as if it were one big vein. Therefore, the RA pressure nearly equals the RV pressure and the PA pressure, with hardly any pulse pressure.

Ventricular tachycardia is a common feature of this disorder, and it may lead to the patient's demise. It is possible that the patient's symptoms of dyspnea and hemoptysis are due to pulmonary embolization emanating from the right heart. Carcinoid syndrome sometimes presents with a thickened, restricted tricuspid valve with regurgitation and/or stenosis. These are associated with higher than normal velocities across the tricuspid valve. This is not tricuspid atresia, because in tricuspid atresia the right ventricle is rudimentary (and here it is enlarged). The tricuspid valve can also be seen to be opening in Figure Q65.1B. Behçet's syndrome is unrelated to this clinical picture.

Somewhere else in this book is a case of massive RV infarction with a similar tricuspid flow pattern.

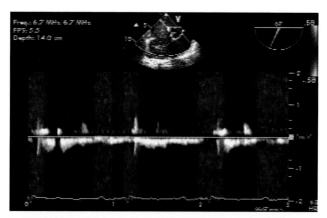

Figure A65.2: Continuous wave Doppler through the tricuspid valve.

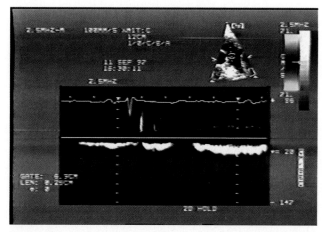

Figure A65.3: Transthoracic echocardiogram, pulsed Doppler of pulmonary artery flow.

> ### *TAKE-HOME LESSON:*
> **Although in this case the RV abnormality is dramatic, the RV should be examined carefully in every patient with ventricular tachycardia, since RV dysplasia may be localized and more subtle.**

66 An Old Starr–Edwards Valve

*F*ifteen years ago this 67-year-old man had mitral valve replacement with a
Starr–Edwards ball and cage prosthesis. He is now complaining of dyspnea
on exertion. On physical examination there are normal prosthetic valve sounds
and a short systolic murmur audible at the left sternal border and the apex.
There was atrial fibrillation but no signs of congestive heart failure. The blood
pressure was 150/90. Transthoracic echocardiography was performed.

This echo showed normal left ventricular function and a normal diastolic flow
velocity pattern across the prosthetic valve (no mitral stenosis). A color Doppler
flow signal was noted (Figure Q66.1).

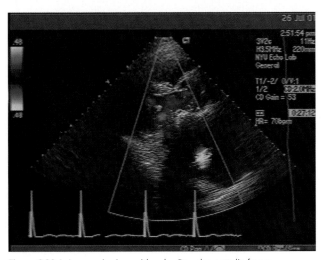

Figure Q66.1: Long-axis view with color Doppler, systolic frame.

QUESTION 66.1. Based on this information, what
would be your next step?

1. Ignore the color Doppler finding
2. Cardiac catheterization with left ventricular
   angiography
3. Transesophageal echocardiography (TEE)
4. Coronary angiography followed by mitral valve
   replacement

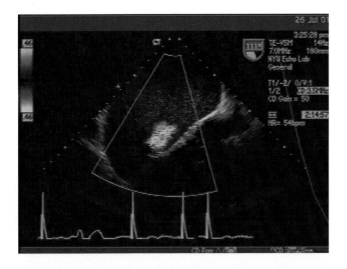

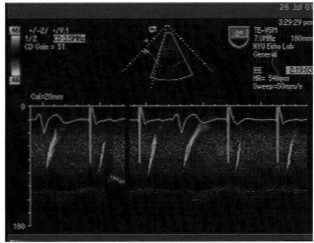

Figure Q66.2D: M-color Doppler of the same flow.

QUESTION 66.2. The patient underwent TEE (Figures Q66.2A through Q66.2D). Note that on some beats, the systolic flow in the left atrium travels to the back of the atrium. Based on this new information, what would you advise now?

1. Ignore the color Doppler finding
2. Cardiac catheterization with left ventricular angiography
3. Magnetic resonance imaging
4. Coronary angiography followed by mitral valve replacement

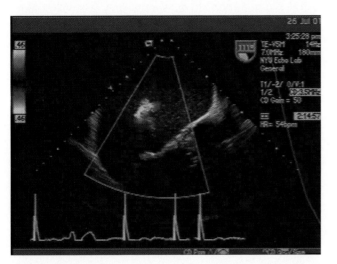

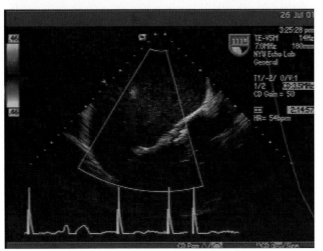

Figures Q66.2A-Q66.2C: Three consecutive systolic frames from the TEE.

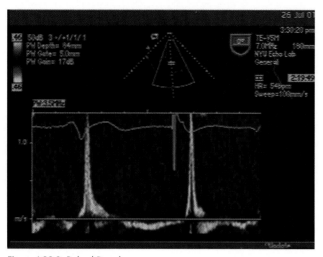

Figure A66.2: Pulsed Doppler.

ANSWER 66.1. The answer is 3, TEE. This is the correct answer, because some of the mitral regurgitation may be masked by the prosthesis on transthoracic echo. It is very possible that although the color signal of mitral regurgitation (MR) seen in the left atrium in Figure Q66.1 is small, the actual degree of MR may be severe. Every patient with a mechanical mitral prosthesis and symptoms should be considered a candidate for TEE for the reason that transthoracic echocardiography may miss severe MR in such patients.

ANSWER 66.2. The correct answer is 1, ignore the color Doppler finding. The TEE shows what is expected when a small volume of blood is displaced toward the left atrium by the ball in the cage. This is not pathological mitral regurgitation. It represents only a small volume that (unlike pathologic mitral regurgitation) moves at a slow velocity. Figure A66.2 shows pulsed Doppler of the same signal. Note that the duration of the signal is short and the velocity is only 1.5 m/second.

TAKE-HOME LESSON:

Not every patient with a prosthetic valve and dyspnea has prosthetic valve malfunction. Always do a TEE if a patient has a mechanical mitral prosthesis and you suspect that it is not working correctly. Nearly every mechanical mitral prosthesis will produce a signal in the left atrium in systole. One has to distinguish between physiologic and pathologic signals.

67 What Did You Bring Back From Nepal?

*T*his 63-year-old male just returned from a trip to Nepal. Last week he had three transient ischemic attacks. The physical examination is entirely within normal limits, and a carotid ultrasound was normal. Transthoracic echocardiography was of poor quality, and a transesophageal echocardiogram (TEE) was performed (Figure Q67.1A).

Did you get it? If not, Figure Q67.1B is a zoomed view.

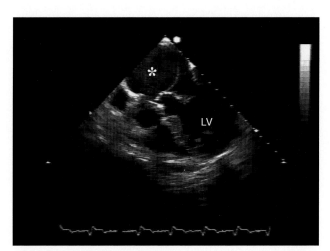

Figure Q67.1A: TEE, four-chamber view.

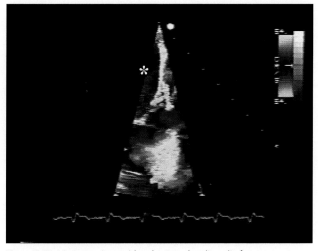

Figure Q67.1C: Same view, with color Doppler, diastolic frame.

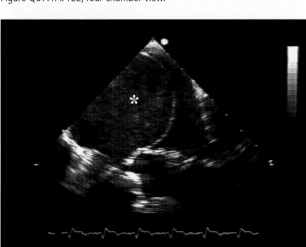

Figure Q67.1B: Closer view of Figure Q67.1

QUESTION 67.1. Note that there is no color flow within the structure marked with an asterisk in Figure Q67.1C. What is this structure?

1. Echinococcal cyst
2. Sinus of Valsalva aneurysm
3. The right atrium
4. Loculated pericardial fluid
5. Inguinal hernia

QUESTION 67.2. What is the source of emboli?

1. Aorta
2. Left atrium
3. Mitral valve
4. Pulmonary vein

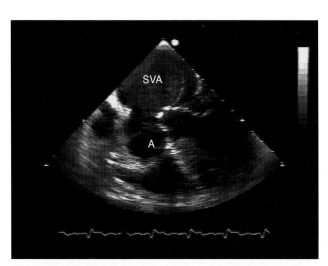

Figure A67.1: TEE, five-chamber view. SVA = sinus of Valsalva aneurysm; A = aortic root.

ANSWER 67.1. The answer is 2, sinus of Valsalva aneurysm. If you selected echinococcal cyst, you must have been influenced by the travel history. However, an echinococcal cyst is a complex structure with septations and "daughter" cysts. In Figure A67.1, a slightly different transducer angle shows the communication between the structure and the aortic root, and therefore this is a rather large sinus of Valsalva aneurysm.

ANSWER 67.2. The answer is 1, embolization from the aorta (sinus of Valsalva aneurysm). This is the likely source of embolization, as there is stagnation within the aneurysm (see spontaneous contrast, noted earlier). The blood in the left atrium does not have such contrast (the flow in the atrium is high, as can be seen on the color Doppler), and is therefore less likely to clot. The pulmonary veins are not obstructed by this aneurysm, and there is no tumor or thrombus on the mitral valve.

TAKE-HOME LESSON:
People who go to Nepal usually return with diarrhea, not with echinococcal cysts.

CASE

68 Complications of Thymoma

A 42-year-old man had a known thymoma that had always been asymptomatic. He was admitted to the emergency room in shock. His blood pressure was 80/45. There was no paradoxical pulse. He had marked jugular venous distention. His oxygen saturation was 88%. A Swan–Ganz catheter was inserted, and the pulmonary artery (PA) pressure was found to be normal. The cardiac output was 9.2 L/minute. Transthoracic echocardiography (TTE) was nondiagnostic, and a transesophageal echocardiogram (TEE) was performed (Figures Q68.1A through Q68.1D).

QUESTION 68.1. Based on these images, what is the reason for this patient's hypotension?

1. High cardiac output
2. Cardiac tamponade
3. Hypovolemia
4. Pulmonary embolus

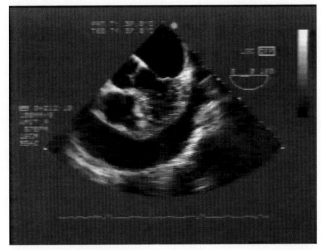

Figure Q68.1A: TEE, 0 degrees.

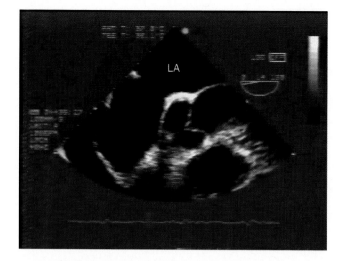

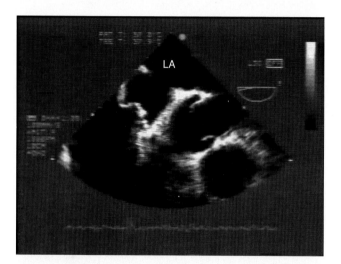

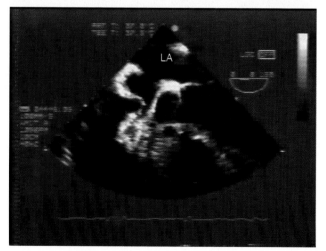

Figures Q68.1B-Q68.D: TEE, three consecutive frames.

The patient also has severe collapse of the right atrium (RA), which is seen in Figures Q68.1B through Q68.1D. The combination of marked RA collapse and large pericardial effusion is highly suggestive of cardiac tamponade. It is unlikely that the patient is hypovolemic as he has severe neck vein distention. It is also unlikely for a patient to develop shock from a pulmonary embolus if he has a normal pulmonary artery pressure. Based on these images, what is the reason for this patient's desaturation?

1. Right-to-left shunt
2. Left-to-right shunt
3. Pulmonary embolus
4. High cardiac output
5. Methemoglobinemia

QUESTION 68.3. Why is the cardiac output high (9.2 L/minute) in this patient with shock?

1. The patient is septic
2. Left-to-right shunt
3. Right-to-left shunt
4. The patient has beriberi and has Graves' disease

QUESTION 68.4. If this patient has cardiac tamponade, why was there no paradoxical pulse?

1. The left ventricular pressures were elevated
2. The patient was hypovolemic
3. Cardiac tamponade compressed only the right ventricle and not the left ventricle
4. The ventricular volumes are fixed throughout the respiratory cycle

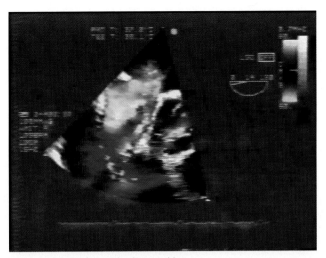

Figure Q68.3A: Left-to-right shunt, in blue.

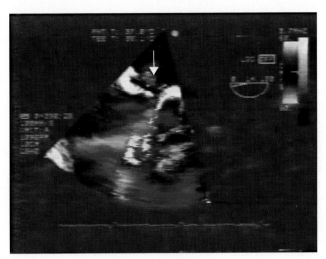

Figure Q68.3B: Right-to-left shunt, in red (arrow).

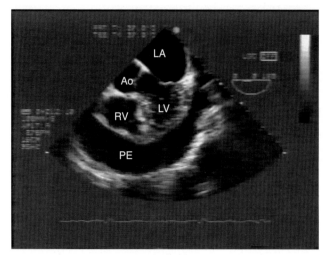

Figure A68.1: Same view as Figure Q68.1A.

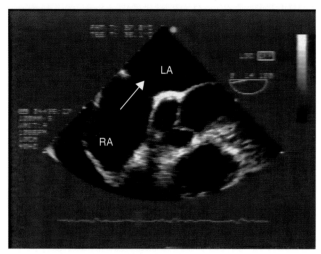

Figure A68.2: Same view as Figure Q68.1B.

ANSWER 68.1. Correct answer: 2, cardiac tamponade. This patient has a large pericardial effusion (PE, Figure A68.1).

ANSWER 68.2. Correct answer: 1, right-to-left shunt. In addition to a pericardial effusion with tamponade, this patient has a large atrial septal defect (ASD; arrow, Figure A68.2).

Cardiac tamponade is responsible for collapse of the RA during diastole, and also occasionally during systole. The collapse that is seen in Figures Q68.1C and Q68.1D empties the RA through the ASD and into the left atrium, resulting in a right-to-left shunt and desaturation. Figure Q68.3A shows the left-to-right shunt in blue when the RA is expanded. Figure Q68.3B shows the right-to-left shunt in red, when the RA is collapsed.

ANSWER 68.3. Correct answer: 2, left-to-right shunt. Note that the "cardiac output" as measured by thermodilution is a measurement of pulmonary blood flow. In spite of the fact that this patient has a right-to-left shunt, most of the shunt is left-to-right, as can be seen by the large blue flow in Figure Q68.3A. The right-to-left shunt occurs only during atrial collapse, which is relatively short. There was no clinical evidence of sepsis, beriberi, or Graves' disease.

ANSWER 68.4. Correct answer: 4, the ventricular volumes are fixed throughout the respiratory cycle. In a patient with an ASD, inspiration increases venous return to the right atrium, and simultaneously decreases the amount of shunt from left-to-right. As a result, the atrial (and also ventricular) volume remains unchanged throughout the respiratory cycle. This is the reason why the second heart sound has fixed splitting in patients with a large ASD.

TAKE-HOME LESSON:

1. **Always think "shunt" if a patient has arterial desaturation.**
2. **Always think shunt if there is a discrepancy between the measured cardiac output and the clinical situation.**
3. **The absence of paradoxical pulse does not rule out tamponade in a patient with an ASD.**

69 Bad Echo From Our Hospital

*T*his is technically the worst echo in this book. It was performed in the recovery room on a 70-year-old patient who had just undergone mitral valve repair. Three years ago, the patient underwent a right pneumonectomy, with a subsequent displacement of the heart. During the mitral repair surgery, the heart could not be visualized by transesophageal echocardiography (TEE), therefore epicardial echo was used for monitoring the procedure. In the recovery room the patient was hypotensive on dobutamine, the pulmonary capillary wedge pressure was 28 mm Hg, and the right atrial pressure was 10 mm Hg. Figure Q69.1 is representative of the only images we could obtain using transthoracic echocardiography (TTE).

QUESTION 69.1. What would you do now?
1. Contrast injection
2. Magnetic resonance imaging (MRI)
3. Computed tomography (CT) with contrast
4. Cardiac catheterization
5. Something else

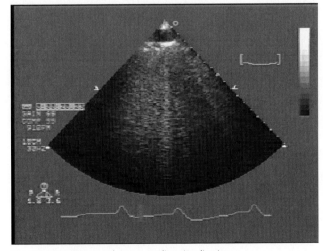

Figure Q69.1: TTE, no adequate cardiac visualization.

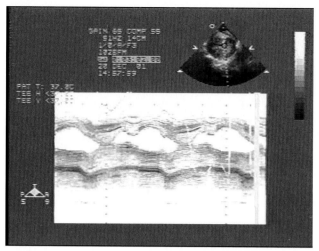

Figure Q69.2A: SEE, M-mode of the left ventricle.

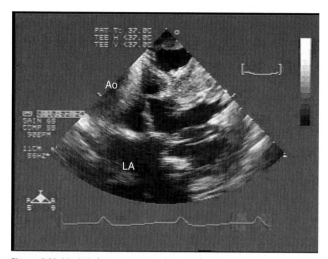

Figure Q69.2B: SEE, long-axis view, diastolic frame.

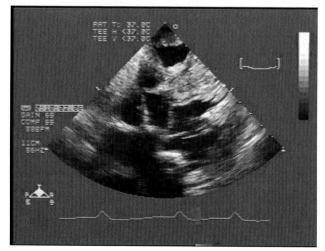

Figure Q69.2C: SEE, long-axis view, systolic frame.

QUESTION 69.2. Knowing that this patient had both a difficult TTE and TEE, the surgeon used this commercially available modified chest tube for mediastinal drainage, and a TEE probe was easily inserted (see Figures A69.1A and A69.1B on next page). Because the probe doesn't come into contact with the body fluids, it doesn't need to be sterile. The images in Figures Q69.2A through Q69.2C were obtained using substernal, epicardial echocardiography (SEE).

There is no consensus on how to present SEE images, but we do them with the anterior structures toward the top and the posterior ones toward the bottom. Therefore the orientation is the opposite of TEE (in the images, the aorta [Ao] is on the left and top of the image; the left atrium [LA] is on the left and bottom).

Based on these images, the treatment should include which of the following?

1. Stop the dobutamine
2. Pericardiocentesis
3. Mitral valve replacement
4. Aggressive diuresis and increase the dose of dobutamine

ANSWER 69.1. Correct answer: 5, something else. (In fact, whenever "something else" is a choice, this is the right answer!) Contrast echocardiography is helpful when you have a poor image, but it is not helpful when there is no window. MRI, CT, and catheterization require moving this critically ill patient out of the recovery room. The correct thing to do is SEE. One other option is intracardiac echocardiography (ICE). However, this requires a special, expensive probe, and it cannot be done on all echo equipment. To perform SEE, a TEE probe is inserted in a modified double-lumen chest tube. One lumen serves as a drain (as a standard substernal chest tube). The other lumen is closed-ended and a TEE probe is inserted into it for cardiac visualization. The tube is shown in Figure A69.1A & A69.1B.

ANSWER 69.2. Correct answer: 1, stop the dobutamine. This patient has developed left ventricular outflow tract (LVOT) obstruction with marked systolic anterior motion (SAM) of the mitral valve. The anterior leaflet can be seen hitting the interventricular septum in systole (Figure A69.2, arrow).

Outflow obstruction due to mitral SAM is a known complication of mitral valve repair with an annuloplasty ring. In this patient the left ventricle (LV) was hyperkinetic, as can be seen in Figure Q69.2A on the M-mode echo. As a result of this, and of the smaller systolic outflow tract size, the flow velocity in the outflow tract is faster. As a result of the faster velocity, the outflow tract pressure is lower (Venturi effect), causing the mitral anterior leaflet to be drawn anteriorly against the septum, obstructing the outflow tract. The large LVOT gradient, which results from this, causes hypotension. There is also reduced systolic coaptation of the mitral valve, leading to mitral regurgitation (raising the left atrial pressure). In most cases, this resolves when inotropes are stopped and the preload is improved (stopping diuretics or giving intravenous fluids).

> ***TAKE-HOME LESSON:***
> 1. **When a patient with a mitral repair is hypotensive, always consider and aggressively look for LVOT obstruction.**
> 2. **SEE is useful in selected patients with no standard echocardiographic windows on TTE and TEE.**

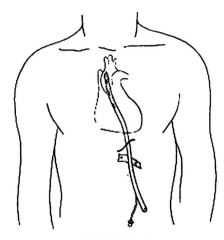

SEE™ Application

Figure A69.1A: SEE, after Hanlon JT, Lowe RI, Funary A. Substernal epicardial echocardiography: A new ultrasonic window to the postoperative heart. *JASE* 2000;13:35–8.

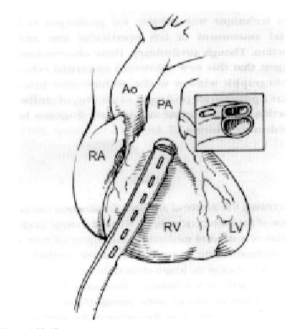

Figure A69.1B

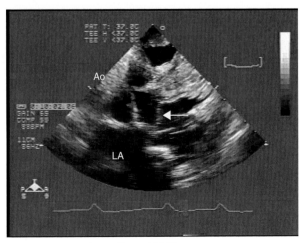

Figure A69.2: Same view as Figure A69.1D.

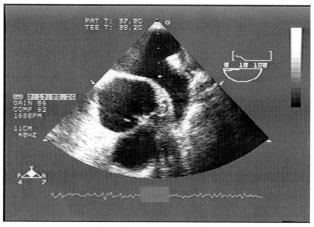

CASE

70 Should You Ligate the Appendage?

This 38-year-old woman had severe mitral regurgitation. She also had a history of paroxysmal atrial fibrillation and one episode of transient aphasia in the past. The following transesophageal echocardiogram (TEE) of the left atrial appendage (Figure Q70.1) was obtained in the operating room, just before mitral valve repair.

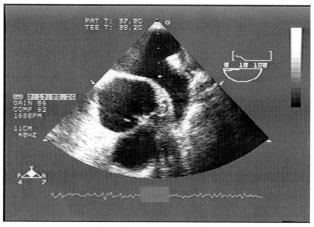

Figure Q70.1: TEE, LA appendage.

QUESTION 70.1. What would you advise the surgeon to do with the left atrial appendage?

1. Leave it alone
2. Ligate it with a line of sutures from the left atrial cavity
3. Amputate it
4. Occlude it with a coil.

156

ANSWER 70.1. Correct answer: 3, amputate it. We and others have observed that nearly 40% of the patients who have an attempt at atrial appendage ligation still have a communication between the appendage and the body of the left atrium (LA). This partial ligation results in a milieu for thrombus formation within the appendage. The partial ligation results in a potential channel for thrombus embolization (see Figure A70.1), as was the case in this patient who returned 1 year after surgery with an embolic stroke.

Figure A70.1 shows a partially ligated left atrial appendage, which contains a thrombus (asterisk). Note that there is blood flow between the appendage and the body of the LA (arrow). The reason for the frequent failure to totally occlude the appendage while suturing from the inside may have something to do with the very shallow bites that the surgeon takes during suturing to avoid the left circumflex coronary artery. Although we, and others, believe that amputation is the correct approach to this problem, others feel that they can occlude the left atrial appendage safely, with no residual communication. More recently, percutaneous techniques for left atrial appendage occlusion have been developed using coils (obviously these would not be used during open heart mitral surgery). In addition, an ablation procedure should be considered in an attempt to prevent further atrial fibrillation.

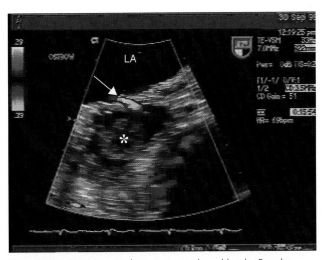

Figure A70.1: TEE, LA appendage, postoperative, with color Doppler.

> *TAKE-HOME LESSON:*
> **Accepted, traditional treatments (surgical and medical) should always be re-evaluated based on newer information.**

CASE

71 Transient Ischemic Attack After Valve Replacement

This 35-year-old woman underwent mitral valve replacement 6 weeks ago. Yesterday she had a brief episode of left-sided weakness. On physical exam, there were crisp valve sounds and a short systolic murmur at the left sternal border. A transesophageal echocardiogram (TEE) was performed (Figures Q71.1A through Q71.1D).

QUESTION 71.1. What type of mitral prosthesis is this?

1. Bjork-Shiley tilting disk
2. Starr-Edwards ball and cage
3. St. Jude's bileaflet tilting disk
4. McGovern-Nixon

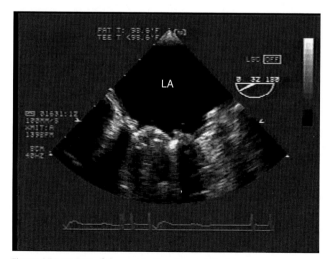

Figure Q71.1A: TEE of the prosthetic valve, systolic frame.

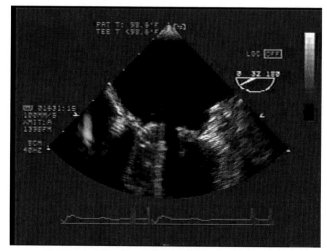

Figure Q71.1B: TEE of the prosthetic valve, diastolic frame.

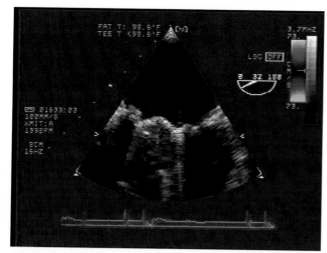

Figure Q71.1C: TEE of the prosthetic valve, with color Doppler, systolic frame.

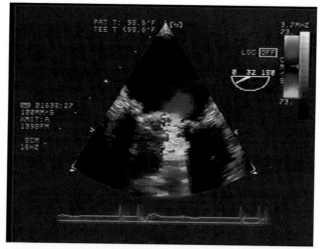

Figure Q71.1D: TEE of the prosthetic valve, with color Doppler, diastolic frame.

QUESTION 71.2. What is wrong with the valve in Figure Q71.2?

1. No problem
2. Abnormal stenosis
3. Abnormal regurgitation
4. One leaflet is stuck
5. 2 and 4 are both correct

QUESTION 71.3. The international normalization ratio (INR) is 3. Magnetic resonance imaging (MRI) of the brain was normal. What would you do now?

1. Watchful waiting (echo in 1 month)
2. Anticoagulation to an INR of 4 to 5.
3. Thrombolysis
4. Surgery

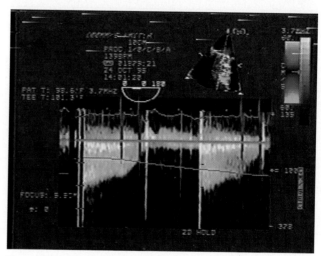

Figure Q71.2: TEE with CW Doppler through the prosthetic valve.

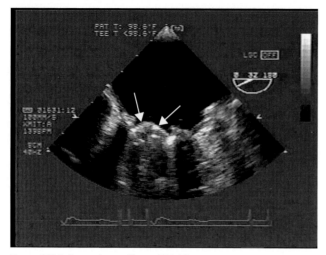

Figure A71.1: Same view as Figure Q71.1A.

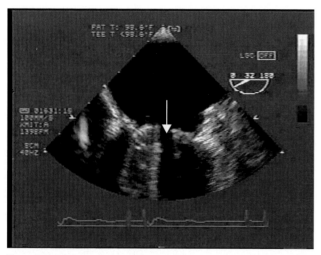

Figure A71.2A: Same view as Figure Q71.1B.

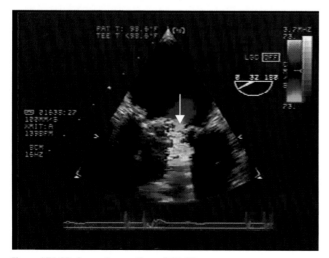

Figure A71.2B: Same view as Figure Q71.1D.

ANSWER 71.1. Correct answer: 3, St. Jude's bileaflet tilting disk. Figure A71.1 clearly shows that there are two disks (arrows). A Bjork-Shiley valve has only one disk. McGovern and Nixon ran for president and did not invent a prosthetic valve (however, there was an unrelated ball-and-cage McGovern prosthesis).

ANSWER 71.2. Correct answer: 5, both 2 and 4 are correct. The diastolic frames in Figures A71.2A and A71.2B show that only one disk is mobile and opens (arrows), and there is flow through this space only, and not on the other side where the disk is stuck in the closed position.

The continuous wave (CW) Doppler in Figure Q71.2 shows that the peak flow velocity across the prosthesis is 2.1 m/second. The mean mitral gradient is 12 mm Hg. The calculated mitral valve area by pressure half time is 1.2 cm^2. These findings are diagnostic of prosthetic mitral valve stenosis. (This is not surprising, because half of the valve is blocked.)

ANSWER 71.3. The correct answer is controversial. What we did was 3, thrombolysis. There was a good result, with restoration of valve function and no complications. On the left side of the heart, there is a risk of embolization resulting from thrombolysis of clots on a prosthesis, and therefore in some centers surgery is preferred. Watchful waiting is not a correct answer in a patient with major prosthetic dysfunction with prosthetic valve stenosis. Anticoagulation to an INR of greater than 4 is potentially dangerous. However, an INR between 3 and 4 has been recommended for patients with a mechanical mitral valve.

72 Endocarditis

*T*his 55-year-old man presented with a 3-day history of fever. Blood cultures were positive for strep viridans. A transesophageal echocardiogram (TEE) is performed, which shows the mitral vegetation pictured in Figures Q72.1A and Q72.1B, as well as severe mitral regurgitation (MR) and a normal left ventricle (LV).

QUESTION 72.1. What would you do?

1. Operate immediately
2. Give intravenous antibiotics until the patient becomes afebrile, and then operate
3. Give intravenous antibiotics until the infection is cured, and then operate (after 6 weeks)
4. Give intravenous antibiotics; if the infection is cured and the patient is asymptomatic, follow the patient medically

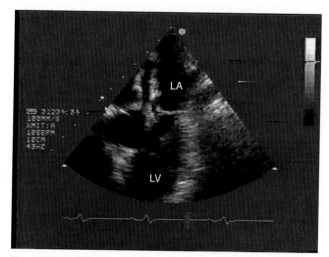

Figure Q72.1A: TEE of the mitral valve, late systolic frame.

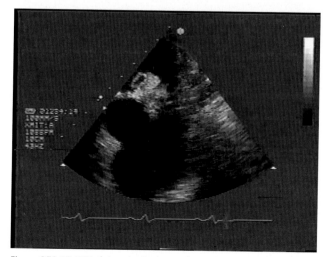

Figure Q72.1B: TEE of the mitral valve, early systolic frame.

ANSWER 72.1. Correct answer: 1, operate immediately. In patients with a mitral vegetation that is larger than 1 to 1.5 cm (and this one is larger than 3 cm!), the risk of embolization before treatment is started is very high (1, 2), and the vegetation should be removed acutely. Because the patient has severe MR, it is very likely that he will have to undergo surgery. Waiting until the operative field has been sterilized poses an unacceptable risk of severe complications, such as stroke.

73 High-Velocity Mitral Regurgitation

*T*he continuous wave (CW) Doppler in Figure Q73.1 was taken on a transthoracic echocardiogam (TTE) through the mitral valve, showing a mitral regurgitation jet that has a velocity of 7.2 m/second. The patient's blood pressure was 120/80.

QUESTION 73.1. Which of the following cannot be the correct diagnosis?

1. High cardiac output
2. Hypertrophic obstructive cardiomyopathy (HOCM)
3. Shone's syndrome
4. Peripheral vascular disease
5. Aortic stenosis

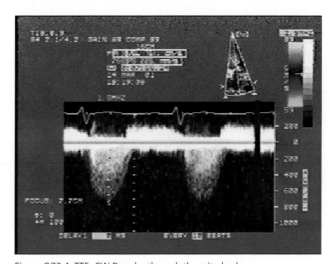

Figure Q73.1: TTE, CW Doppler through the mitral valve.

ANSWER 73.1. Correct answer: 1, high cardiac output. This patient has a very high pressure in the left ventricle, as can be judged by the left ventricle-left atrial (LV–LA) gradient as calculated from the MR jet velocity of 7.2 m/second. Putting this value into the modified Bernoulli equation (Pressure gradient = $4V^2$), the LV–LA gradient is 207 mm Hg. Thus the LV pressure is 207 plus the LA pressure, or about 217 mm Hg (if the LA pressure is 10 mm Hg). Because the blood pressure in the brachial artery is 120, there must be an obstruction between the LV and the brachial artery with a gradient of 217 – 120 = 97 mm Hg. Such a gradient is possible with aortic stenosis, HOCM, Shone's syndrome (multiple obstruction in the left heart, including subvalvular, valvular, and supravalvular atrial stenosis), or peripheral vascular disease with stenosis of an artery proximal to the brachial artery. A high cardiac output will not create a pressure gradient between the LV and the aorta, and therefore the LV pressure will be close to the brachial artery pressure.

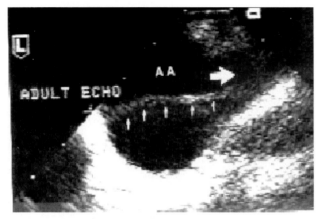

CASE 74 Can You Name This Vessel?

A 73-year-old man underwent a transesophageal echocardiogram (TEE) because of severe chest pain and a murmur of aortic insufficiency. The image in Figure Q74.1 was obtained.

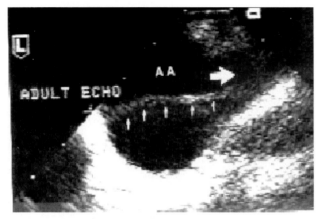

Figure Q74.1: TEE of the aortic arch, 90 degrees.

QUESTION 74.1. Based on this image, what is your diagnosis?

1. Aortic dissection extending into the left carotid artery
2. Aortic dissection extending into the left subclavian artery
3. Aortic dissection extending into the innominate artery
4. No aortic dissection; the line marked with small arrows is an artifact
5. There is no way to tell from this image alone

QUESTION 74.2. Because it is important to decide if the dissection extends into the carotid or into the subclavian, what would you do?

1. Magnetic resonance imaging (MRI)
2. Contrast aortography
3. Doppler
4. Echo contrast
5. Tissue Doppler imaging

164

ANSWER 74.1. Correct answer: 5, no way to tell from this image alone. Figure Q74.1 shows a clear dissection flap (arrows) within the aortic arch. The flap extends into a great vessel, but there is no way to distinguish between the subclavian and the carotid from this image alone. The innominate artery is usually not seen on TEE.

ANSWER 74.2. Correct answer: 3, Doppler. By withdrawing the transducer, the carotid and subclavian can be seen side by side (Figure A74.2A). These two great vessels have a different flow pattern that can be seen on the spectral tracing. Because the carotid supplies the brain, there is a low-resistance pattern (with continued flow in diastole). Because the subclavian artery supplies the skeletal muscles of the area, there is a high-resistance pattern (systolic predominantly, with early diastolic reversal of flow and no flow through the rest of diastole). In Figure A74.2B, in the subclavian (left), flow is nearly all systolic, with a brief early diastolic reversal (typical of a high-resistance vessel). In the carotid (right), flow continues throughout diastole (a low-resistance pattern). In this case, the dissection is into the carotid artery.

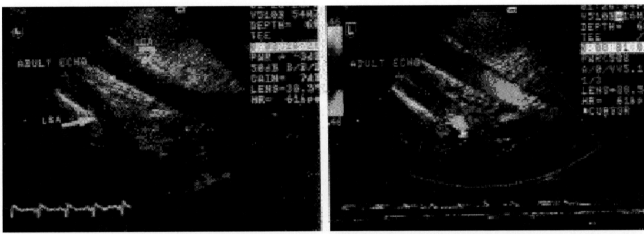

Figure A74.2A: TEE of the carotid and subclavian arteries, with color Doppler, systolic frame.

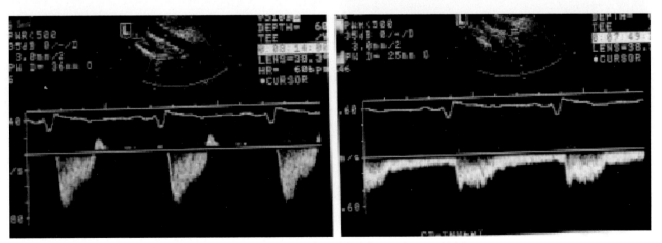

Figure A74.2B: Pulsed Doppler spectral tracings of the left subclavian (left) and the left carotid arteries (right).

CASE

75 How Is This Mitral Regurgitation Different?

A 44-year-old man had an echocardiogram. The spectral tracing in Figure Q75.1 was obtained using continuous wave (CW) Doppler with the transducer at the apex, recording mitral regurgitation (MR).

Based on this tracing, try to answer the following questions.

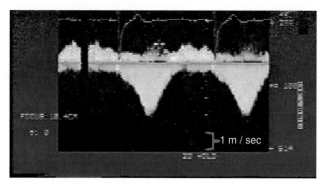

Figure Q75.1: CW of mitral regurgitation.

QUESTION 75.1. Is the patient having a good day?

1. Yes
2. No
3. You can't tell

QUESTION 75.2. What is the left atrial pressure?

1. High
2. Low
3. Normal
4. You can't tell

QUESTION 75.3. What is the left ventricular ejection fraction?

1. High
2. Low
3. Normal
4. You can't tell

QUESTION 75.4. What is the degree of mitral regurgitation?

1. Mild
2. Moderate
3. Severe
4. You can't tell without color Doppler

ANSWER 75.1. Correct answer: 2, no, the patient is not having a good day. See the following explanation.

ANSWER 75.2. The correct answer is 1, the left atrial pressure is high. Because the peak velocity of the mitral regurgitation is about 3 m/second, the left ventrical-left atrial (LV-LA) pressure gradient is about 36 mm Hg ($4V^2$). The reason for this is either an extremely low LV pressure and/or an extremely high LA pressure; more likely, a combination of the two.

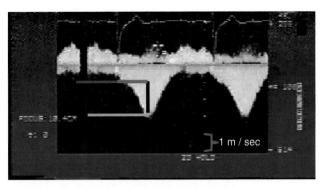

Figure A75.3: Same view as Figure Q75.1.

ANSWER 75.3. The correct answer is 2, the ejection fraction is low. How do we know this from one CW tracing? Note that the rate of rise of the mitral regurgitation jet velocity is slow. The reason for this is the slow rise of systolic pressure in the left ventricle. In other words, the LV dP/dt is low. The dP/dt can be calculated from the CW tracing (Figure A75.3):

The LV-LA pressure gradient at the time that the velocity is 1 msec (red line) is 4 mm Hg. The LV-LA pressure gradient at the time that the velocity of MR is 3 m/second (green line) is 36 mm Hg. The time that it takes for the LV-LA pressure to rise from 4 mm Hg to 36 mm Hg (the time that it takes to rise 32 mm Hg) is the length of the blue line, or 150 m/second (this is dt). Therefore dP/dt (the change in pressure per 1000 msec) is (32 / 150) × 1000, or 213 mm Hg/second. The normal value is about 800 mm Hg/second. Therefore, this patient has a very low LV dP/dt, the most important marker of contractility. The ejection fraction is therefore very low.

ANSWER 75.4. The correct answer is 3, severe. The pixel density of the MR jet is the same as that of the mitral diastolic inflow. This indicates that within the sample volume, a large quantity of blood is moving in the wrong direction in systole. This patient therefore has a high LA pressure and a low LV pressure, with severe MR and a severely hypokinetic LV. He is in cardiogenic shock, and cannot be having a good day.

TAKE-HOME LESSON:
One spectral tracing may be worth 1,000 words!

76 Swollen Leg

A 70-year-old man had cardiac catheterization 1 week ago. He now presents with a swollen, ecchymotic, and warm right leg. Although this is a book about noninvasive examination of the heart, the ultrasound test on this patient will examine problems that may arise from the invasive evaluation of the heart (Figures Q76.1A and Q76.1B).

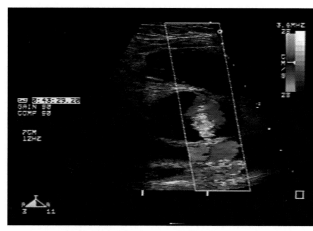

Figure Q76.1A: Right groin study, systolic frame.

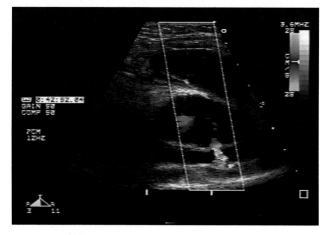

Figure Q76.1B: Right groin study, diastolic frame.

QUESTION 76.1. What happened to this patient?

1. Subcutaneous hematoma
2. Femoral arteriovenous fistula
3. Femoral pseudoaneurysm
4. All of the above (1, 2, and 3) are correct
5. Only 1 and 3 are correct

QUESTION 76.2. How would you treat the patient?

1. Watchful waiting with repeat ultrasound in 1 week
2. External compression with the ultrasound transducer
3. Thrombin injection
4. Surgical repair

ANSWER 76.1. Correct answer: 4: Numbers 1, 2, and 3 are all correct. There are four spaces visualized (Figure A76.1A).

(H) is the hematoma, (P) is the pseudoaneurysm (4 × 3 cm), (A) is the femoral artery, and (V) is the femoral vein. These can all be differentiated by the color flow and spectral pattern and timing. There is no flow at all into the hematoma. There is turbulent flow through a hole in the femoral artery into the pseudoaneurysm in systole (Figure A76.1A, arrow), and lower velocity flow into the femoral artery (out of the pseudoaneurysm) in diastole (seen in Figure A76.1B, arrow). Thus, the flow is to-and-fro between the artery and the pseudoaneurysm, diagnostic of a pseudoaneurysm (see also Figure A76.1C).

This patient has two perforations in his right femoral artery. The anterior perforation leads to a collection of blood (a pseudoaneurysm). The posterior perforation leads into the adjacent femoral vein. Note the high-velocity turbulent flow both anteriorly (into the pseudoaneurysm) and posteriorly (into the vein).

The flow from the femoral artery into the femoral vein is seen both in systole and diastole. Although the velocity is higher during systole, the direction is the same in both systole and diastole (as opposed to the flow into the pseudoaneurysm). The flow into the vein through the fistula is shown in Figure A76.1D.

To better distinguish between the two pathologic flows from the femoral artery, a zoomed view with a different transducer, is shown in Figure A76.1E.

ANSWER 76.2. Correct answer: 4, surgical repair. This is what we have done with this patient. Watchful waiting may be recommended for small pseudoaneurysms. However with this size lesion, and with the addition of a symptomatic AV fistula, this is not advised. External compression is a fairly benign therapy for pseudoaneurysms. However it is less successful for AV fistulae. In addition, the presence of the large hematoma superficial to the

lesions makes it less likely that this will be successful. We tried it, and we couldn't even stop the blood flow into the pseudoaneurysm. Thrombin injection is now considered to be the treatment of choice for an isolated pseudoaneurysm. However, it would have no effect on the AV fistula, and in fact it could cause venous thrombosis.

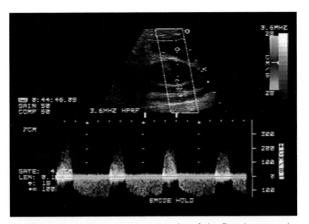

Figure A76.1C: Continuous wave Doppler of the flow between the artery and the pseudoaneurysm.

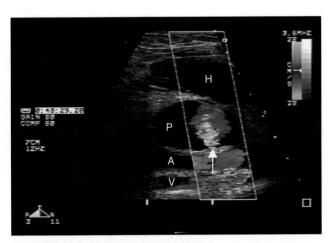

Figure A76.1A: Same view as Figure Q76.1A.

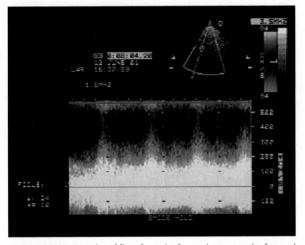

Figure A76.1D: Doppler of flow from the femoral artery to the femoral vein (AV fistula).

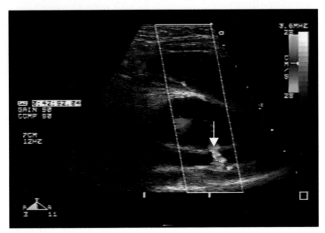

Figure A76.1B: Same view as Figure Q76.1B.

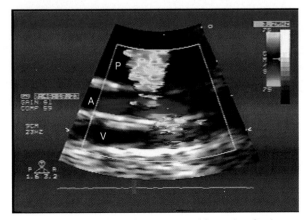

Figure A76.1E: Femoral pseudoaneurysm and femoral AV fistula, systolic frame, zoomed view.

77 Is This What They Taught You in Medical School?

A 67-year-old woman was referred for echocardiography because of palpitations. She was found to be in atrial flutter.

The sonographer noticed that something was not right, and showed you the M-mode tracing in Figure Q77.1).

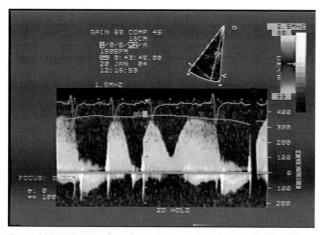

Figure Q77.1: CW Doppler echocardiogram of aortic valve flow.

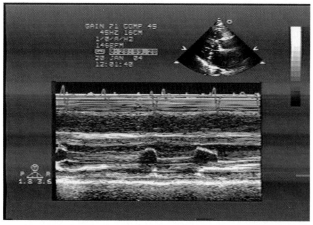

Figure Q77.2: M-mode echo of the mitral valve.

QUESTION 77.1. What went wrong?

1. The echo machine
2. Con Edison
3. The sonographer pushed the wrong button
4. The patient

QUESTION 77.2. However, this patient also had other abnormalities of flow. Study Figure Q77.2 carefully and try to answer the next question.

Which of the following may also be present?

1. Holodiastolic mitral regurgitation
2. Systolic mitral stenosis
3. Diastolic aortic stenosis
4. All of the above

ANSWER 77.1. Correct answer: 4, the patient. After the second QRS, the patient has aortic insufficiency both in systole and diastole. After the second QRS, left ventricular pressure did not reach the aortic pressure, and therefore the aortic valve did not open and there was no antegrade aortic flow. Aortic regurgitation continued into systole. This is seen again, even better, after the third QRS. For these two beats (second and third) there was also no antegrade flow through the aortic valve, and therefore no pulse (pulse deficit). You've already seen this earlier in this book.

Therefore, this part was easy.

ANSWER 77.2. Correct answer: 1, Holodiastolic mitral regurgitation. Figure Q77.2 shows that the mitral valve does not open before the second QRS. This means that the left ventricular pressure remained higher than the left atrial pressure throughout the cardiac cycle (including diastole!). This is the substrate for holodiastolic mitral regurgitation. Note the pulsed Doppler of mitral flow in Figure A77.2A. This suggests that the left ventricular pressure is higher than the left atrial pressure throughout the cardiac cycle, because there is no diastolic flow before the second QRS.

Continuous wave (CW) Doppler (Figure A77.2B) shows that indeed there is continuous mitral regurgitation throughout systole and diastole between the second and third QRS, and again between the sixth and the ninth QRS.

The M-mode color Doppler in Figure A77.2C shows that mitral regurgitation (green mosaic color) continues throughout systole and diastole before and after the second QRS. Note that there is no antegrade flow (in red) seen before the second QRS.

Not convinced yet that there may be holodiastolic mitral regurgitation? The tissue Doppler of the lateral mitral annulus is shown in Figure A77.2D. Note that the mitral ring velocity is away from the transducer (below the baseline) during diastole and toward the transducer in systole-but not for the third QRS (arrow). Before that beat, the annulus does not move away from the left ventricular apex, meaning that the ventricle does not fill on that beat. In systole, the annulus does not move toward the apex (and the transducer), meaning that the ventricle does not empty. This is proof that when the mitral valve doesn't open in diastole, the aortic valve also does not open on the following systole.

Figure A77.2E shows the same story with the tricuspid valve.

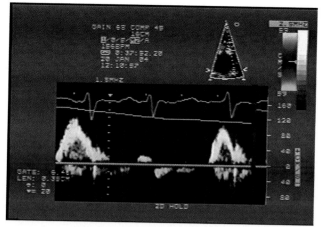

Figure A77.2A: Pulsed Doppler of mitral flow.

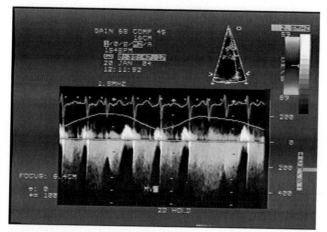

Figure A77.2B: CW Doppler of mitral flow.

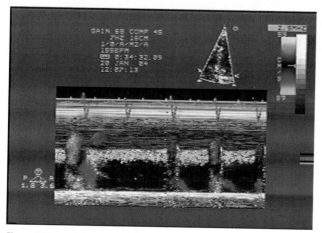

Figure A77.2C: Color M-mode Doppler of mitral flow.

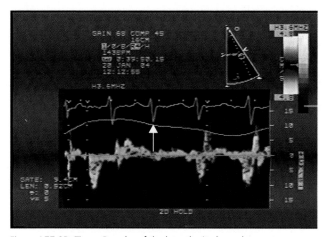

Figure A77.2D: Tissue Doppler of the lateral mitral annulus.

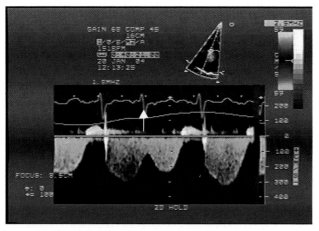

Figure A77.2E: CW Doppler of tricuspid valve flow.

Note that there is holodiastolic tricuspid regurgitation before the second QRS, and that the tricuspid valve does not open (there is no forward flow) before the second QRS (arrow).

Figure out for yourself what happened with the pulmonic valve (not shown out of pity).

TAKE-HOME LESSON:

Contrary to what they taught you in medical school, mitral and tricuspid regurgitation may be holodiastolic, and aortic and pulmonic regurgitation may be holosystolic!

78 Was It a Successful Operation?

A 27-year-old asymptomatic female had minimally invasive cardiac surgery for closure of a secundum atrial septal defect (ASD). The heart was approached via a small right thoracotomy, and the atrial septum was approached through an incision in the right atrial wall. At the end of the surgery, intraoperative transesophageal echocardiogrphy (TEE) was interpreted as showing an intact repair (Figure Q78.1). After surgery, the patient developed dyspnea. Cyanosis and hemoglobin desaturation (oxygen saturation equals 70% by pulse oximetry) were then noted.

Note that no shunting is seen between the atria.

QUESTION 78.1. Spiral computed tomography (CT) scanning showed no evidence of pulmonary emboli, and Doppler did not show any evidence of pulmonary hypertension. What would you do now?

1. Right heart catheterization
2. Buy a new oximeter
3. Repeat echo with saline injection into the left arm
4. Repeat echo with saline injection into the right leg
5. Check methemoglobin level

QUESTION 78.2. What happened?

1. The patient had undetected Scimitar syndrome
2. The surgeon performed a Glenn procedure by mistake
3. The surgeon closed the wrong hole by mistake
4. The echo was done on the wrong patient

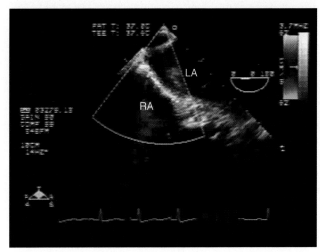

Figure Q78.1: Immediate postoperative TEE.

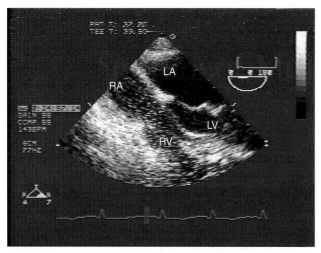

Figure A78.1A: TEE 0 degrees, modified four-chamber view, with left-arm saline injection.

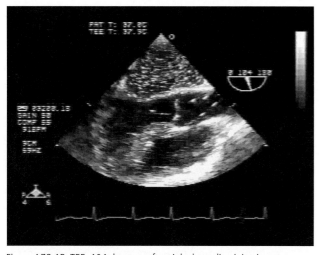

Figure A78.1B: TEE, 104 degrees, after right-leg saline injection.

ANSWER 78.1. Correct answer: 4, repeat echo with saline injection into the right leg. To be honest, we reached this conclusion by trial and error. Let us share it with you. Knowing that there was no pulmonary hypertension, we didn't think that right heart catheterization would add any additional information. We first tried a left-arm saline injection to explore the possibility of an unusual venous communication (for example, a persistent left superior vena cava may have an unusual drainage, not only into the right atrium via the coronary sinus, but if the coronary sinus is "unroofed," into the left atrium). The left arm saline injection appears in Figure A78.1A.

Note that microcavitations appear in the right heart, but not in the left heart, excluding a right-to-left shunt with this injection. We even checked for methemoglobinemia, which was not present.

Figure A78.1B shows what happened after injection of saline into the right femoral vein.

ANSWER 78.2. Correct answer: 3, the surgeon closed the wrong hole by mistake. The diagrams in Figures A78.2A and A78.2B explain what happened.

The surgeon placed a patch between the eustachian valve and the superior margin of the ASD. This diverted all of the (unoxygenated) inferior vena cava (IVC) blood into the left atrium, causing the patient's oxygen desaturation.

Figure A78.2C confirms the new anatomic condition.

Note the communication with the left atrium (LA).

In the fetus, the eustachian valve (which is anatomically located at the inferior margin of the IVC) serves to divert blood from the lower half of the body, across the interatrial septum. In this case, it did the same thing (thanks to the "repair"), but this was detrimental.

TAKE-HOME LESSON:

Murphy's law holds true, even in cardiac surgery and echocardiography. If something can go wrong, it will.

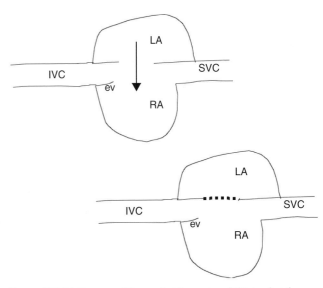

Figures A78.2A: Diagram of the surgical "procedure." This is what the surgeon thought he was doing: closing an ASD with a patch (dotted line).

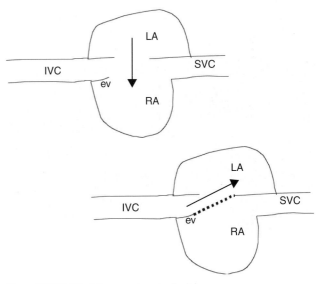

Figure A78.2B: What the surgeon actually did.

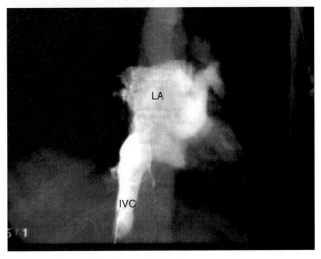

Figure A78.2C: Dye injection into the IVC.

79 The Patient Who Fell From Her Bed

A 79-year-old woman fell from her bed. She was taken to the emergency room, complaining of back pain that increased with inspiration. A transesophageal echocardiogram (TEE) was performed to rule out cardiac or aortic damage. The heart was normal, and there was no pericardial effusion. The findings in the thoracic aorta are shown in Figures Q79.1A through Q79.1C.

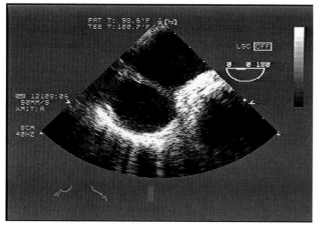

Figure Q79.1A: TEE of the proximal descending thoracic aorta, 0 degrees.

QUESTION 79.1. Based on these findings, what would you do?

1. Do more testing
2. Treat the descending aortic dissection with a stent
3. Treat the descending aortic dissection medically
4. Change the machine settings, you are seeing an artifact

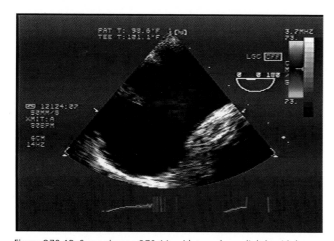

Figure Q79.1B: Same view as Q79.1A, with transducer slightly withdrawn.

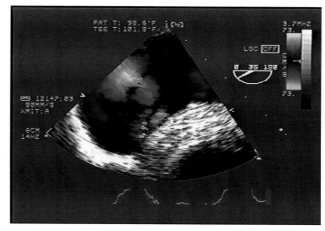

Figure Q79.1C: 35-degree view, with color Doppler.

ANSWER 79.1. Correct answer: 1, do more testing. This is not likely to be a dissection, because the apparent flap is perpendicular to the aortic wall. Also, there does not appear to be separation of the blood flow into true and false lumens on color Doppler. Although traumatic transection remains in the differential diagnosis, the flap in a transection is frequently very mobile (see the video for Case 79). Linear artifacts are frequently seen in the aorta on TEE. However, they are usually vague and can be traced outside of the aortic image, unlike what was seen in this case. Here there is a discrete finding within the aorta, and this is not an artifact.

The direction of the descending aorta in these horizontal views is unusual (normally it appears as a circle). This indicated tortuosity of the descending aorta. To further evaluate this patient, a magnetic resonance angiogram (MRA) was ordered (Figure A79.1.).

Note the markedly tortuous descending aorta. A kink is noted (arrow). This was imaged by the TEE, and gave the false impression that there was a flap present. The patient had rib fractures, with no traumatic damage to the aorta.

TAKE-HOME LESSON:

Atypical findings on TEE need confirmation by other imaging modalities before emergency surgery is contemplated.

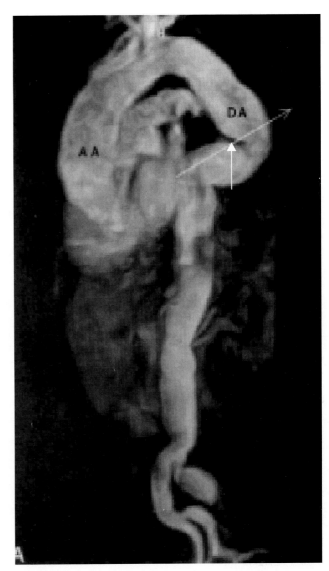

Figure A79.1: MRA of the thoracic aorta.

80 Fever of Undetermined Origin

A 37-year-old woman had fever of up to 101°F for 3 weeks. Her erythrocyte sedimentation rate (ESR) was markedly elevated (102 mm/hour). There were no murmurs on examination, and the transthoracic echo was unremarkable. Transesophageal echocardiography (TEE) was performed to rule out endocarditis (Figures Q80.1A through Q80.1C). The valves were normal.

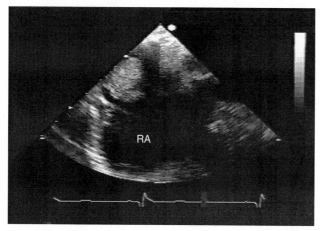

Figure Q80.1A: TEE at a depth of 40 cm, 0 degrees, showing the right atrium.

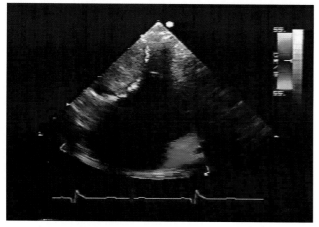

Figure Q80.1B: Same view, with color Doppler.

QUESTION 80.1. Based on these findings, what is the most likely diagnosis?

1. Acute massive pulmonary embolism
2. Constrictive pericarditis
3. Right atrial myxoma
4. Extracardiac tumor
5. Sarcoidosis

QUESTION 80.2. Based on these images and the clinical syndrome, what is the most likely diagnosis?

1. Hypernephroma
2. Adrenal carcinoma
3. Benign uterine leiomatosis
4. Thymoma

QUESTION 80.3. Immediately after the TEE, the patient went into shock, and the electrocardiogram (EKG) showed marked repolarization changes. What would you do now?

1. Call a gastroenterologist to rule out an esophageal perforation or massive bleeding
2. Repeat the TEE
3. Arrange for urgent coronary angiography
4. Right heart catheterization (Swan-Ganz).

QUESTION 80.4. Now what is the correct diagnosis?

1. Bleeding or esophageal perforation
2. Massive pulmonary embolus
3. Acute myocardial infarction (MI)
4. Sepsis

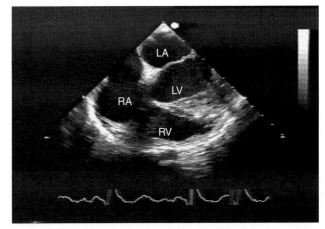

Figure Q80.1C: Modified four-chamber view, 0 degrees.

ANSWER 80.1. Correct answer: 4, extracardiac tumor.

In Figure A80.1, note that the inferior vena cava (IVC) is markedly dilated and filled with a tumor mass (Tu). The mass is outlined by the turbulent color flow. Acute massive pulmonary embolism is usually associated with a dilated right ventricle (RV) (and the RV is normal in Figure Q80.1C). A right atrial myxoma is usually attached to the interatrial septum, and rarely is it on the wall of the right atrium (RA). It is never in the IVC. There is nothing on these images to suggest either of the other two diagnoses (constrictive pericarditis or sarcoidosis).

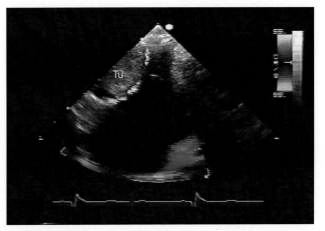

Figure A80.1: Same view as Figure Q80.1B.

ANSWER 80.2. Correct answer: 1, hypernephroma. This tumor is coming from below the diaphragm, and fills the IVC. Therefore it cannot be a thymoma. Because there is a fever of unknown origin and a very high ESR, hypernephroma is the most likely diagnosis, and that's what it was.

ANSWER 80.3. Correct answer: 2, repeat the TEE. A representative image appears in Figure A80.3.

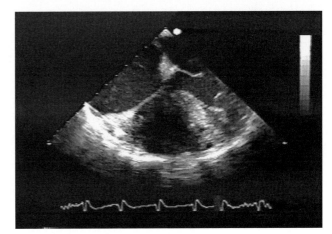

Figure A80.3: Same TEE view as in Figure Q80.1C.

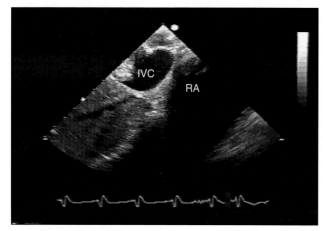

Figure A80.4A: TEE of the IVC and the RA.

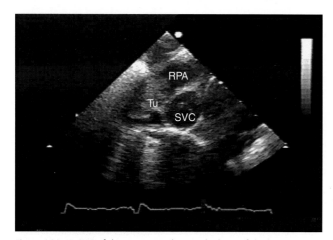

Figure A80.4B: TEE of the great vessels near the base of the heart.

ANSWER 80.4. The cause of the patient's hemodynamic decompensation is seen in Figures A80.4A and A80.4B.

Note that there is a large piece of the tumor missing from the IVC in Figure A80.4A (compare this with the IVC in Figure Q80.1). This piece is now lodged in the right pulmonary artery (RPA), as seen in Figure A80.4B (Tu). In spite of resuscitation attempts, the patient expired. An autopsy revealed a hypernephroma extending into the IVC, with a large tumor embolus to the lung.

TAKE-HOME LESSON:

Always remember that a TEE is not a totally benign procedure. It is possible that the gagging and coughing in this patient, and possibly even the direct pressure of the transducer, may have led to this lethal pulmonary tumor embolism.

CASE

81 Ascites

A 62-year-old man with myeloid metaplasia received radiation to the chest 2 years ago for suspected myeloid infiltration of the pericardium. He developed exercise intolerance, peripheral edema, and ascites. On examination, the blood pressure was 100/60 with a 15 mm Hg paradoxical pulse. There was massive ascites and a tender, enlarged liver as well as marked lower extremity edema. The Doppler tracing of his mitral inflow is shown in Figure Q81.1.

QUESTION 81.1. Based on this Doppler tracing, what is the least likely diagnosis?

1. Pericardial effusion with tamponade
2. Constrictive pericarditis (fibrosis)
3. Compression of the heart by a tumor
4. Infiltrative, restrictive cardiomyopathy

QUESTION 81.2. Figures Q81.2A through Q81.2D are from his transthoracic echo.

Based on these images, what is the most likely diagnosis?

1. The diagnosis cannot be made from the echo
2. Hepatoma
3. Cardiac sarcoma
4. Cardiac lymphoma
5. Fibrosis

QUESTION 81.3. What would you recommend now?

1. Radionuclide study
2. Magnetic resonance imaging (MRI)
3. Computed tomography scan
4. Contrast angiography
5. Positron emission tomography scan

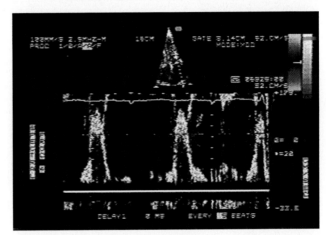

Figure Q81.1: Pulsed Doppler of transmitral flow.

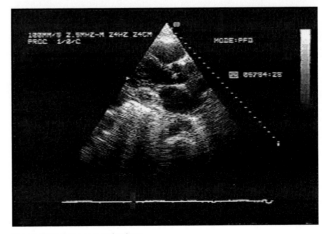

Figure Q81.2A: Long-axis view.

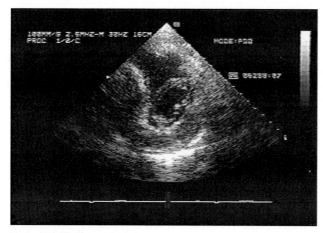

Figure Q81.2B: Short-axis view.

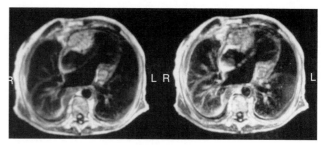

Figure A81.3: MRI with and without gadolinium.

ANSWER 81.1. Correct answer: 1, Pericardial effusion with tamponade. This is the only entity listed that does not have rapid ventricular filling and a rapid deceleration time. In this patient, the deceleration time was 120 m/second (normal ≥ 160 m/second). Respiratory variation (present in constriction but not in restriction) would be helpful here, but it is not visible on this short tracing.

ANSWER 81.2. Correct answer: 1, the diagnosis cannot be made from the echo. There is clearly a mass that is compressing both the right ventricle (RV) and the left ventricle (LV), and this is responsible for the constrictive hemodynamics seen in Figure Q81.1 and this patient's symptoms. However, echocardiography is not a good tool for tissue characterization and can not distinguish among different pathologies.

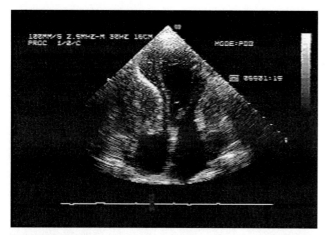

Figure Q81.2C: Four-chamber view.

ANSWER 81.3. Correct answer: 2, MRI. With gadolinium, tumors will enhance and fibrosis will not. In this patient there was no enhancement (Figure A81.3), making fibrosis the most likely diagnosis. Because of the patient's symptoms, he underwent surgery where massive fibrosis was documented and treated. There were no neoplastic cells found, and all cultures were negative. After surgery, all of the patient's symptoms disappeared.

Note that the mass is on either side of the left ventricle (LV) and that it does not enhance with gadolinium.

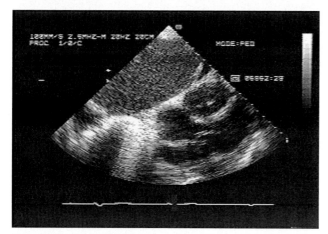

Figure Q81.2D: Subxiphoid view.

82 Right Atrial Mass After Surgery

A 52-year-old man underwent triple coronary artery bypass grafting 11 years ago. He returns now because of chest discomfort. His workup included echocardiography that showed no wall motion abnormalities, and the finding seen in Figures Q82.1A and Q82.B.

QUESTION 82.1. Based on these images, what would you do first?

1. Ignore the finding, it's a normal variant
2. Do a transesophageal echocardiogram (TEE)
3. Do coronary angiography
4. Do magnetic resonance imaging (MRI)

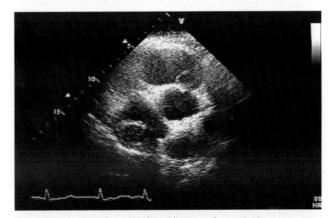

Figure Q82.1A: Transthoracic echocardiogram, short-axis view.

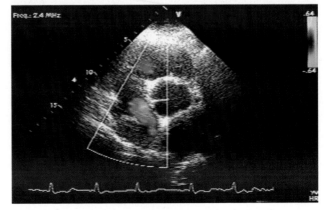

Figure Q82.1B: Same view as Figure Q82.1A, with color Doppler.

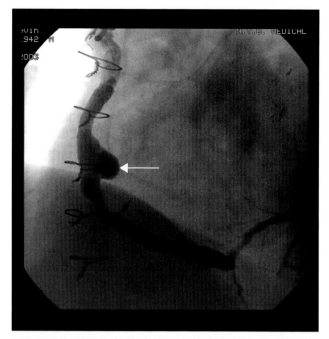

Figure Q82.2: Angiogram of the right coronary saphenous vein graft.

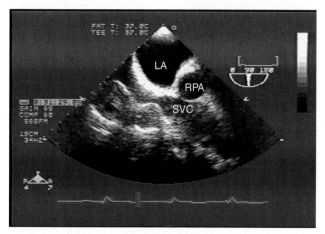

Figure A82.1: TEE, bicaval view (90 degrees).

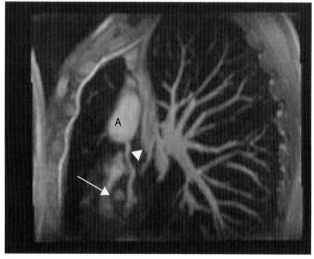

Figure A82.2: MRA.

ANSWER 82.1. We did answer 2 first, a TEE. However, as will be seen next, each of these modalities supported the correct diagnosis. Although mass-like normal or benign variants may occasionally be seen in the right atrium (such as a eustachian valve, a Chiari network, pectinate muscles, internodal pathways, a lipomatous interatrial septum, or a prominent tricuspid annulus), this mass is approximately 3 cm in diameter and unlikely to be a normal variant. Therefore a TEE was done. Except for the mass seen in Figure A82.1, the TEE was unremarkable.

Note the snowman-like bilobed mass in the right atrium, with a maximum short-axis diameter of 3.5 cm. Because of the history of chest pain, and the prior bypass surgery, coronary angiography was then performed. The left coronary grafts were patent and unremarkable.

QUESTION 82.2. Note that there is a localized aneurysmal dilatation of the vein graft (arrow, Figure Q82.2). The maximal diameter of the aneurysm is 9 mm.

Why is the diameter of the aneurysm on angiography much smaller than the diameter on the echo?

1. The finding on the echo represents a different lesion
2. The lesion shrank between the echo and the angiogram
3. Measurements on angiography are misleading
4. There is clot around the lumen of the aneurysm

ANSWER 82.2. Correct answer: 4, there is clot around the lumen of the aneurysm. This was proven with magnetic resonance angiography (MRA), seen in Figure A82.2.

Here, A = aorta; arrow head = saphenous vein graft; arrow = complex aneurysm of the vein graft. Note that the contrast appears within the aneurysm as two round lumens (one on each side of the center). The entire aneurysm is much bigger, and appears as a dark shadow, containing clot.

TAKE-HOME LESSON:

Angiograms are "lumen-o-grams," and therefore they may not show the entire size of vessels. Echocardiography and MRI show the entire size of the vessel. The fact that flow was not demonstrated within the aneurysm on color Doppler may be related to low flow velocity and to the small size of the lumen, which could have been missed.

83 I Had Surgery

*T*his 74-year-old man came to the emergency room with severe shortness of breath. He had a history of heart surgery 1 year ago but could not recall any of the details. The images in Figures Q83.1A to Q83.1D are from an echocardiogram obtained in the emergency room.

QUESTION 83.1. What is the most likely reason for this patient's mitral regurgitation?

1. Posterior leaflet perforation
2. Degeneration of a tissue prosthesis
3. Anterior leaflet mitral prolapse
4. Dehiscence of a mitral annuloplasty ring
5. Mitral orifice clot

QUESTION 83.2. Prior to surgery, this patient had normal coronary arteries and left ventricular wall motion. On this echocardiogram, there is akinesis of the base of the posterior wall and the lateral wall. What is the most likely reason for this?

1. Long pump time
2. Newly developed atherosclerotic coronary occlusion
3. Coronary artery ligation
4. New left bundle branch block (LBBB)

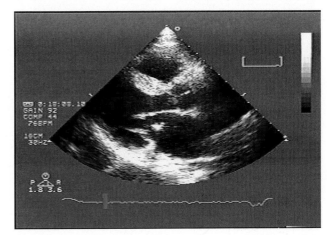

Figure Q83.1A: Long-axis view.

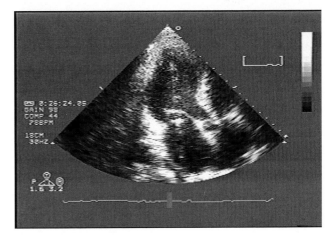

Figure Q83.1B: Two-chamber view.

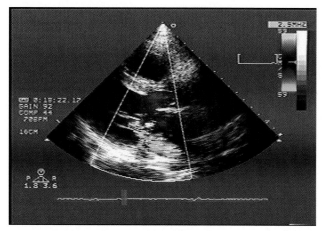

Figure Q83.1C: Long-axis view with color Doppler.

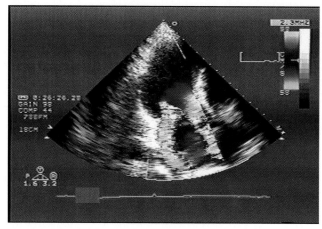

Figure Q83.1D: Two-chamber view with color Doppler.

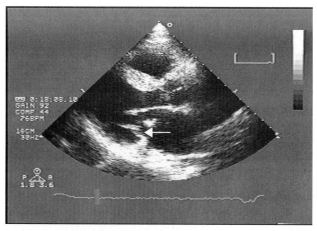

Figure A83.1: Same view as Figure Q83.1A.

ANSWER 83.1. Correct answer: 4: dehiscence of a mitral annuloplasty ring. This patient had undergone a mitral valve repair using an annuloplasty ring. Figure Q83.1A shows a space between the posterior aspect of the annuloplasty ring and the mitral annulus (arrow).

Thus there is a jet of mitral regurgitation that is between the mitral leaflets, but outside (behind) the dehisced ring.

ANSWER 83.2. Correct answer: 3, coronary artery ligation. Ligation of the circumflex artery is a known, unfortunate complication of suturing the posterior part of the annuloplasty ring. The proximal circumflex is located in the left atrioventricular groove, just behind the posterior suture line.

84 Transient Ischemic Attack One Month After Surgery

*T*his 62-year-old man had severe coronary artery disease and severe mitral regurgitation, as well as severe chronic obstructive pulmonary disease (COPD). It was felt that mitral valve replacement with coronary artery bypass surgery posed an unacceptable risk, and therefore a different procedure was performed. Initially the patient did well, but 1 month later he had transient aphasia and the following transthoracic echo was performed (Figure Q84.1).

QUESTION 84.1. What operation did the patient have?

1. Endoscopic mitral valve repair
2. Coapsys device
3. Exclusion of a left ventricular aneurysm
4. Alfieri procedure

QUESTION 84.2. Figures Q84.1 and Q84.2 show the cause of the patient's transient ischemic attack (TIA). What is the reason for the TIA?

1. Intracardiac clot
2. Mitral valve endocarditis
3. Aortic atheroma
4. Patent foramen ovale

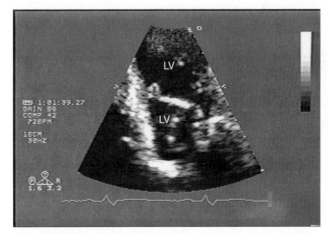

Figure Q84.1: Four-chamber view.

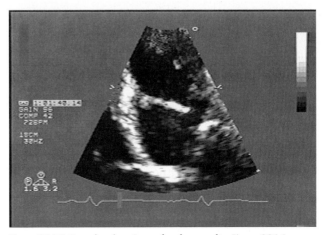

Figure Q84.2: Four-chamber view, a few frames after Figure Q84.1.

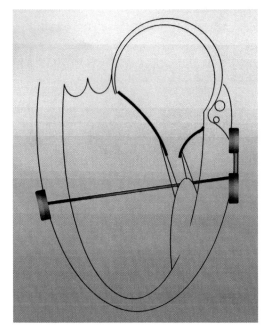

Figure A84.1: Coapsys device.

ANSWER 84.1. Correct answer: 2, Coapsys device. New procedures that are being developed to repair the mitral valve less invasively are accompanied by new echocardiographic findings that will have to be recognized by future echocardiographers. In this patient a dense line is seen traversing the left ventricular cavity just distal to the mitral leaflets. This is a Coapsys device (Myocor, Maple Grove, Minnesota), which has been inserted into the left ventricle in order to change the geometry of the mitral ring to prevent mitral regurgitation. The device is inserted into the left ventricle without opening it, and therefore it does not require the use of cardiopulmonary bypass. Although the technique is still experimental, initial results are encouraging.

The mitral valve is not visualized here (it is masked by the device), and although the mitral valve can be repaired endoscopically, sometimes using the Alfieri procedure (which sutures the mitral leaflet tips to prevent prolapse). Exclusion of a left ventricular aneurysm does not address the issue of mitral regurgitation.

ANSWER 84.2. Correct answer: 1, intracardiac clot. A clot has formed on the Coapsys device (Figure A84.2A, arrow). It is mobile, as can be seen from its movement from above the device in Figure A84.2A to below the device in Figure A84.2B.

The other answers represent common reasons for embolic events, but they are not visualized on the images.

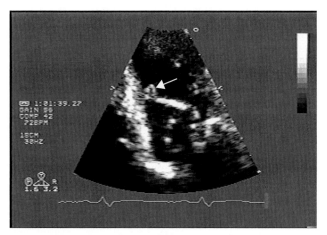

Figure A84.2A: Same view as Figure Q84.1.

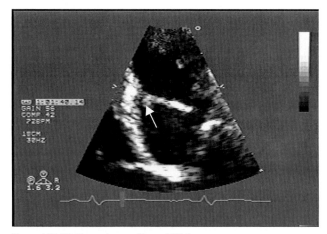

Figure A84.2B: Same view as Figure Q84.2.

85 Twenty-Four-Pound Weight Gain

*A*n 80-year-old man presented with dyspnea and wheezing. He was treated with bronchodilators, but improved only slightly. The following echocardiogram was performed.

The velocity of early diastolic flow (E) in Figure Q85.1A (arrow) is approximately 90 cm/second, and the velocity of the early diastolic wall motion (e') in Figure Q85.1B (arrow) is approximately 5 cm/second.

QUESTION 85.1. Does the patient have asthma, and what is the left atrial (LA) pressure likely to be?

1. Yes: it is approximately 5 mm Hg
2. Yes: it is approximately 12 mm Hg
3. No: it is approximately 22 mm Hg
4. No: it is approximately 35 mm Hg

QUESTION 85.2. What does the M-mode echo in Figure Q85.2 tell you?

1. The patient has a low pulmonary artery pressure
2. The patient has a low left atrial pressure
3. The patient has a low aortic pressure
4. The patient has a low stroke volume

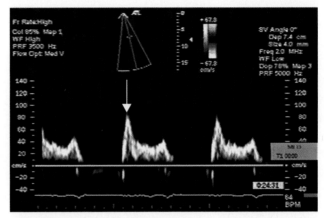

Figure Q85.1A: Pulsed Doppler of mitral inflow.

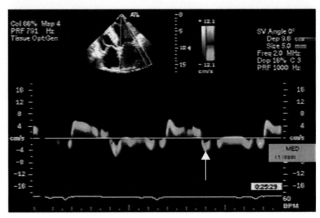

Figure Q85.1B: Tissue Doppler of the lateral mitral annulus.

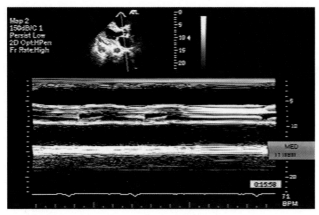

Figure Q85.2: M-mode of the aorta and left atrium.

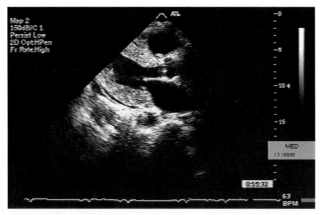

FigureQ85.3: Long-axis view.

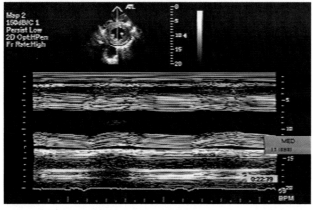

Figure A85.3: M-mode of the right and left ventricles.

QUESTION 85.3. Based on Figure Q85.3, what will the electrocardiogram (EKG) show?

1. High voltage
2. Low voltage
3. Wolff-Parkinson-White syndrome
4. Right axis deviation

ANSWER 85.1. Correct answer: 3, no, it is approximately 22 mm Hg. The LA pressure can be estimated by dividing the mitral E velocity on pulsed Doppler by the early diastolic (e') velocity on tissue Doppler, and adding 4 mm Hg. Pulsed Doppler shows a "restrictive pattern" with a high E and low As with a rapid deceleration time.

ANSWER 85.2. Correct answer: 4, the patient has a low stroke volume. The normal early diastolic reduction of left atrial size (with ventricular filling) is absent. In fact, there is little or no reduction in LA size throughout diastole. This indicates one of two things-the patient has either mitral stenosis, or a low stroke volume with a low volume of atrial emptying (ventricular filling) throughout diastole.

ANSWER 85.3. Correct answer: 2, low voltage. The left ventricle (LV) wall thickness is increased (approximately 2 cm), and most patients with this finding will have high voltage left ventricle hypertrophy on EKG. However, the bright appearance of the myocardium and the trace pericardial effusion are hints that what the patient really has is amyloidosis, which will produce a low voltage QRS (the amyloid has replaced the myocardium). In this case, the patient had senile (transthyretin) amyloid. This disease may present with dramatic fluid accumulation, as it did in our patient. Amyloidosis (or less common causes or restrictive cardiomyopathy) should be strongly considered when the echocardiogram shows increased wall thickness and the EKG shows low voltage.

Figure A85.3 shows the reduction in systolic function (ejection fraction) caused by the patient's amyloidosis.

Note the thick LV walls and reduced systolic excursion (the ejection fraction was approximately 20%).

TAKE-HOME LESSON:

Wheezing is not always asthma! The LA pressure can be estimated from the Doppler examination (mitral inflow and tissue velocity), and left ventricular failure can be ruled in or ruled out as a cause of wheezing or dyspnea.

C A S E

86 A Tough Decision

A 73-year-old man had two myocardial infarctions, 15 and 5 years ago. Four years ago he underwent triple coronary artery bypass surgery. At that time, he had only mild aortic stenosis. He now complains of angina on minimal exertion. Echocardiography was performed (Figures Q86.1A through Q86.1D).

The peak aortic gradient is 31 mm Hg, and the mean gradient is 19 mm Hg. The peak velocity of the left ventricle outflow tract (LVOT) is 60 cm/second.

QUESTION 86.1. Based on these data, what is the severity of the aortic stenosis?

1. Mild
2. Moderate
3. Severe
4. Need more data

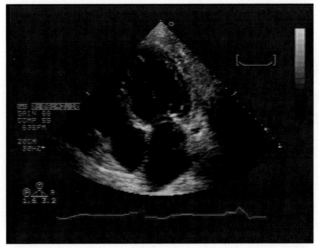

Figure Q86.1A: Transthoracic echocardiogram, apical four-chamber view, diastolic frame.

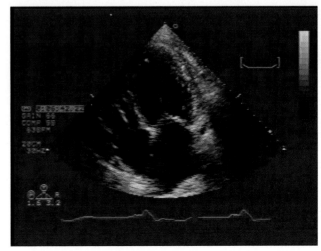

Figure Q86.1B: Same view as Figure Q86.1A, systolic frame.

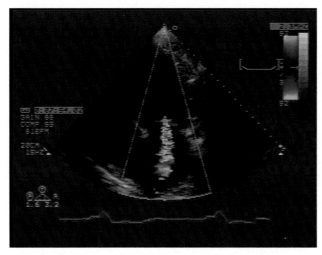

Figure Q86.1C: Same view as Figure Q86.1A, with color Doppler.

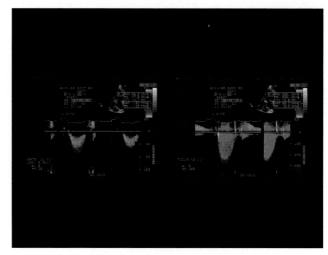

Figure Q86.1D: Doppler echocardiogram: LVOT (left) and aortic valve (right).

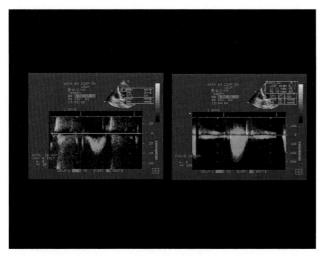

Figure Q86.2: Doppler echocardiogram (LVOT, left; aortic valve, right) at peak dobutamine infusion.

QUESTION 86.2. The peak aortic gradient on dobutamine was 31 mm Hg and the mean gradient was 21 mm Hg (Figure Q86.2). The peak LVOT velocity was 55 cm/second.

Coronary angiography showed total left main coronary occlusion, a patent left internal mammary artery graft to the left anterior descending coronary artery, a patent saphenous vein graft to the circumflex coronary artery, a patent saphenous vein graft to the diagonal, and a new severe midright coronary artery stenosis (the right coronary artery was not bypassed).

Based on these results, what would you recommend now?

1. Aortic valve replacement with right coronary artery bypass
2. Aortic valve replacement, mitral valve repair, and coronary artery bypass
3. Aortic valve replacement, and recheck the degree of mitral regurgitation after the aortic valve is replaced; repair the mitral valve only if the mitral regurgitation (MR) is still significant; coronary artery bypass
4. Right coronary artery stenting
5. Medical therapy

ANSWER 86.1. Correct answer: 4, need more data. The peak velocity of the transaortic valve flow is 2.8 m/second (because the peak gradient is 31 mm Hg, and peak gradient equals 4 (v^2). Thus the dimensionless ratio of transaortic flow velocity: LVOT flow velocity is 4.7. Values over 4 indicate a severely reduced valve area. In this patient, the aortic valve area by continuity was 0.7 cm². However, in patients with low-gradient aortic stenosis (AS) and poor left ventricle function, increased transvalvular flow (during dobutamine infusion, for example) may open the valve more. Therefore, the severity of AS can not be determined from a single resting study. The patient subsequently underwent dobutamine stress echocardiography. There was no change in left ventricular wall motion or ejection fraction.

ANSWER 86.2. Correct answer: 4, right coronary artery stenting. Although it is tempting to want to replace the aortic valve, repair the mitral valve, and bypass the coronary obstruction, this procedure would have an unacceptable mortality rate for this patient. In one study, the in-hospital mortality rate for aortic valve replacement in the presence of an average ejection fraction of 21% due to prior myocardial infarction was 45%. The 6-month mortality was 60%. In this patient with two large scars from prior infarctions, without evidence of viability (no improvement of wall motion and stroke volume on dobutamine), the best approach would be to treat the symptom of angina with right coronary artery stenting. After this was discussed with the patient and his family, he underwent this procedure, and improved. His prognosis remains guarded.

*S*ix weeks ago, this 57-year-old woman underwent an aortic valve replacement with a tissue prosthesis. Two weeks ago she began to complain of fever and fatigue. She then presented to the emergency room with pulmonary edema. Her blood pressure was 70/50. Transthoracic echocardiography (TTE, not shown) was of poor quality, but it suggested good left ventricular function. Transesophageal echocardiography (TEE) was performed (Figures Q87.1A through Q87.1C).

QUESTION 87.1. What is the diagnosis?

1. Atrial septal defect with right-to-left shunt
2. Mitral valve perforation with mitral regurgitation
3. Left ventrical-left atrial (LV-LA) paravalvular communication (fistula)
4. Aorta-LA paravalvular communication (fistula)
5. Prosthetic aortic regurgitation

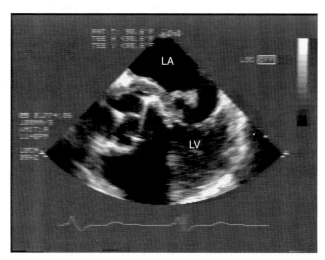

Figure Q87.1A: TEE showing the LA, LV, and the aortic prosthesis (0 degrees).

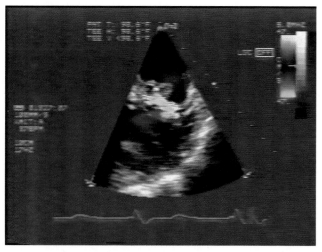

Figure Q87.1B: Same view as Figure Q87.1A, with color Doppler.

QUESTION 87.2. Based on the information that you have, what is the pressure in the left atrium during ventricular systole and diastole?

1. 54 mm Hg in systole, 25 mm Hg in diastole
2. 25 mm Hg in systole, 54 mm Hg in diastole
3. 16 mm Hg in systole, 16 mm Hg in diastole
4. You cannot calculate the left atrial pressure without knowing the gradient across the aortic valve

ANSWER 87.1. Correct answer: 4, Aorta-LA paravalvular communication (fistula).

From Figure Q87.1B, it can be seen that the jet enters the left atrium (therefore 5 is not correct). There is a paravalvular aortic abscess (Figure A87.1, asterisk) behind the prosthesis, with fistula formation that leads to the left atrium. A vegetation is also seen (Figure A87.1, arrow). There is a color jet of flow from around the aortic prosthesis curving upward (in red) into the left atrium.

The continuous wave Doppler in Figure Q87.1C shows that the flow into the left atrium is continuous throughout systole and diastole, suggesting that the communication is originating in the aorta (and not the left ventricle, which would produce a mitral regurgitation jet only in systole).

ANSWER 87.2. Correct answer: 1, the left atrial pressure is 54 mm Hg in systole, 25 mm Hg in diastole. The pressure in the atrium equals the aortic pressure minus the aorta-left atrial (Ao-LA) gradient (you don't need to know the gradient across the aortic valve because you are dealing with the pressure in the aorta beyond the aortic valve). Therefore, in systole the pressure in the LA is the systolic blood pressure (70) minus the systolic gradient between the aorta and the LA. The continuous wave Doppler shows that the flow velocity in systole is 2 m/second; therefore the aorta-left atrial gradient in systole is 16 mm Hg and the left atrial pressure is therefore 70 – 16 = 54 mm Hg). During diastole, the flow velocity is 2.5 m/second; therefore the diastolic gradient is 25 mm Hg and the diastolic left atrial pressure is 50 – 25 = 25 mm Hg. With such a high left atrial pressure, it is no wonder that the patient is in pulmonary edema.

It is surprising that the aorta-left atrial pressure gradient is lower in systole than in diastole, even though the aortic pressure is higher in systole than in diastole. This is because the left atrial pressure is much higher in systole because of the shunt (which although continuous, is much larger in systole) Also, in diastole the mitral valve is open and the left atrial pressure is lower.

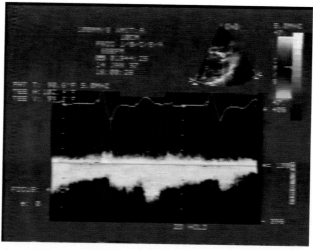

Figure Q87.1C: Continuous wave Doppler obtained during TEE, of the color jet seen in Figure Q87.1B.

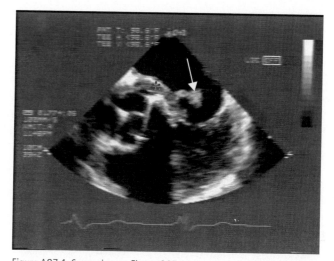

Figure A87.1: Same view as Figure Q87.1A.

88 Dyspnea in Pregnancy

*T*his 24-year-old woman from eastern Europe is now in the second trimester of her first pregnancy. Two weeks ago she started to complain of dyspnea, which has now increased to the point where she can not climb one flight of stairs. On examination there was a diastolic rumble at the apex and a systolic ejection murmur at the base. An echocardiogram was ordered, however the transthoracic echo (TTE) was technically suboptimal (Figures Q88.1A through Q88.1D).

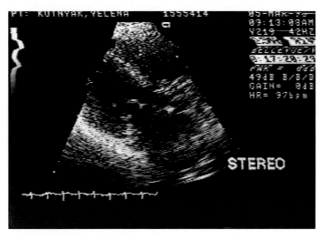

Figure Q88.1A: Long-axis view.

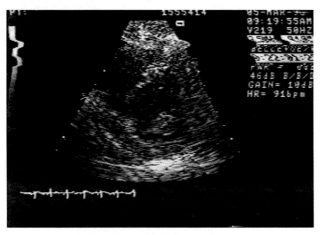

Figure Q88.1B: Short-axis view of the left ventricle.

QUESTION 88.1. Based on these images, the most likely etiology for this patient's problem is which of the following?

1. Congenital
2. Rheumatic
3. Systemic lupus erythematosus
4. Peripartum cardiomyopathy

QUESTION 88.2. To further evaluate this patient, transesophageal echocardiography (TEE) was performed (Figures Q88.2A-D).

The main reason for the patient's high left ventricular outflow velocity (seen in Figure Q88.1D) is which of the following?

1. Subvalvular aortic stenosis
2. Valvular aortic stenosis
3. Supravalvular aortic stenosis
4. All of the above

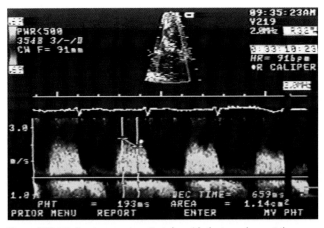

Figure Q88.1C: Continuous wave Doppler with the transducer at the apex, recording left ventricular inflow (scale in msec).

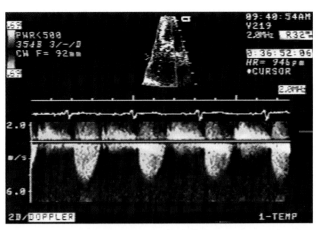

Figure Q88.1D: Continuous wave Doppler with the transducer at the apex, recording left ventricular outflow (scale in msec).

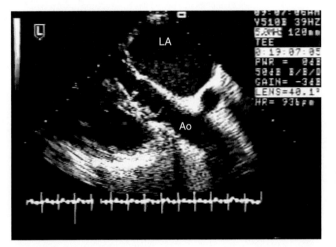

Figure Q88.2A: TEE, 90-degree view.

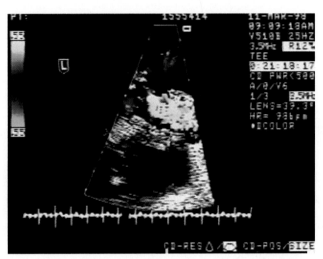

Figure Q88.2B: TEE, same view as Figure Q88.2A, with color Doppler.

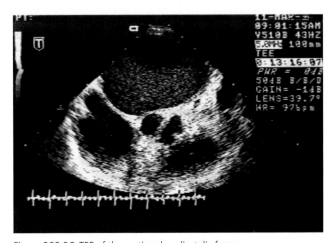

Figure Q88.2C: TEE of the aortic valve, diastolic frame.

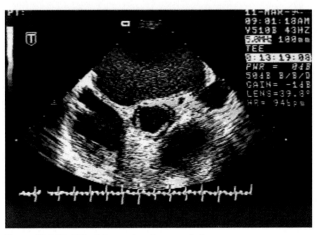

Figure Q88.2D: TEE of the aortic valve, systolic frame,

QUESTION 88.3. Based on these images, what is the severity of the valvular bicuspid aortic stenosis?

1. Mild
2. Moderate
3. Severe
4. Cannot tell

QUESTION 88.4. What is the name of the syndrome that this patient has?

1. Williams' syndrome
2. Turner syndrome
3. Holt-Oram syndrome
4. Shone syndrome

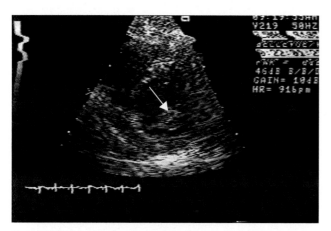

Figure A88.1: Same view as Figure Q88.1B.

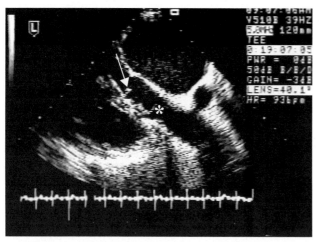

Figure A88.2: Same view as Figure Q88.2A.

ANSWER 88.1. Correct answer: 1, congenital. This patient has significant mitral and aortic stenoses (the mitral valve area calculated by pressure half-time in Figure Q88.1C is 1.1 cm² and the peak aortic gradient [Figure Q88.1D] is 64 mm Hg with a measured mean gradient of 40 mm Hg). Although most mitral stenoses are rheumatic in origin, this one does not appear to be rheumatic. Figure Q88.1A shows relatively thin mitral leaflets without the characteristic commissural fusion that would have indicated a rheumatic etiology. Figure Q88.1B shows that there is only one papillary muscle, and therefore this patient has a congenital parachute mitral valve (Figure A88.1, arrow).

ANSWER 88.2. Correct answer: 4, all of the above. Figure A88.2 shows that there is a subvalvular aortic membrane (arrow). The doming, bicuspid aortic valve is marked by an asterisk. In addition, the ascending aorta is hypoplastic (1.3 cm at its narrowest point, just above the valve). This ascending aortic narrowing is, by itself, an obstruction to flow.

ANSWER 88.3. Correct answer: 4, cannot tell. Although in Figure Q88.2D it looks as though the aortic valve area is normal, one has to remember that the bicuspid aortic valve is doming open in systole, and therefore this cut may not represent the narrowest opening of the valve.

ANSWER 88.4. Correct answer: 4, Shone syndrome. Williams' syndrome patients have supravalvular aortic stenosis (and elfin facies). Turner's syndrome patients have aortic coarctation (and XO genotype). The Holt-Oram syndrome consists of atrial septal defect and mesocardia (with skeletal abnormalities). The Shone syndrome was first described in 1963, and it includes multiple stenoses including coarctation, subaortic stenosis, supravalvular aortic stenosis, and parachute mitral valve. Not all four obstructions are necessarily significant, or even present. Our patient also had a partial supravalvular mitral ring, as shown in Figure A88.4 (arrow).

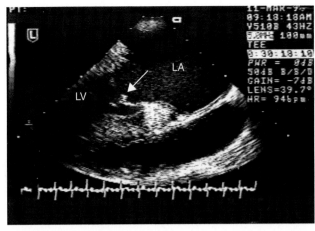

Figure A88.4: TEE, 90 degrees.

89 Pulmonary Artery Compression

*T*he patient is an 87-year-old man who was admitted because of chest and abdominal pain and weakness. His blood pressure was 100/70. The following day the patient became tachypneic and diaphoretic, and had severe abdominal pain. Echocardiography was performed (Figures Q89.1A through Q89.1C). There was normal left ventricular function. The tricuspid regurgitation velocity was normal (2.5 msec).

To assess the flow velocity across the pulmonic valve, a continuous wave Doppler was performed.

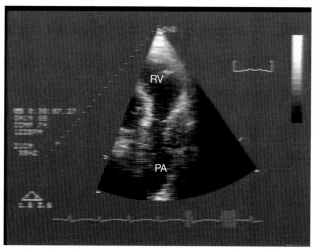

Figure Q89.1A: Subxiphoid view of the right ventricular infundibulum and the pulmonary artery.

QUESTION 89.1. Based on the Doppler in Figure Q89.1C, what is the diagnosis?

1. Valvular pulmonic stenosis
2. External compression of the right ventricular infundibulum
3. Coronary artery fistula into the pulmonary artery
4. Left-to-right shunt
5. Patent ductus arteriosus

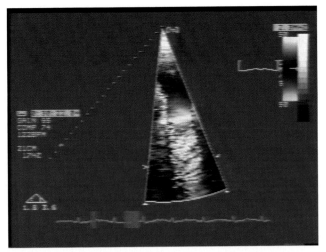

Figure Q89.1B: Same view as Figure Q89.1A, with color Doppler.

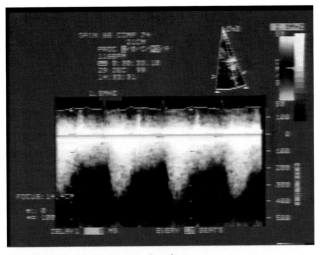

Figure Q89.1C: Continuous wave Doppler.

QUESTION 89.2. The patient went to surgery, and the following direct epicardial echo was obtained.

Based on Figures Q89.1A through Q89.1C and this new information, what is the diagnosis?

1. Atrial septal defect (ASD)
2. Ventricular septal defect (VSD)
3. Ruptured ascending aortic aneurysm into the main pulmonary artery
4. Ruptured descending aortic aneurysm into the left pulmonary artery
5. Left-ventricle-to-right-atrium shunt

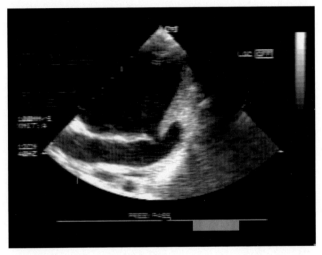

Figure Q89.2A: Direct epicardial echo.

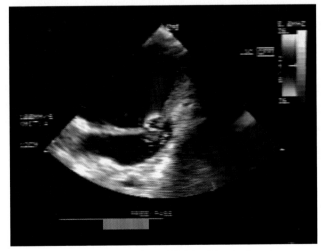

Figure Q89.2B: Same view as Figure Q89.2A, with color Doppler.

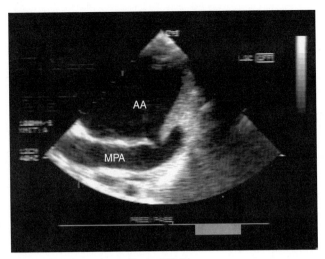

Figure A89.2: Same view as Figure Q89.2A.

ANSWER 89.1. Correct answer: 4, left-to-right shunt. Although there appears to be some external compression of the right ventricular infundibulum, this did not produce a large gradient because right ventricular systolic pressure (as estimated from the velocity of tricuspid regurgitation) is not elevated. Therefore the 4 m/second flow velocity seen in Figure Q89.1C is not because of valvular pulmonic stenosis or external compression of the right ventricular infundibulum. The reason for the turbulent flow in the pulmonary artery seen in Figure Q89.1B must be something else. A coronary artery fistula into the pulmonary artery will produce a higher velocity in diastole than in systole (because the pulmonary artery diastolic pressure is lower than the systolic pressure) and the velocity in a coronary artery fistula will not reach such a high velocity as is seen here (4 m/second in systole and 2 m/second in diastole). A patent ductus arteriosus may have the flow pattern seen here in Figure Q89.1C, however the flow will be in the opposite direction (i.e., from the left pulmonary artery toward the pulmonic valve and the transducer, above the baseline).

ANSWER 89.2. Correct answer: 3, ruptured ascending aortic aneurysm into the main pulmonary artery.

In Figure Q89.2A, a hole is seen, and in Figure Q89.2B one can clearly see a proximal isovelocity surface area (PISA) indicating flow acceleration as blood moves from a high-pressure chamber to a lower pressure chamber. Along with the fact that the flow acceleration can be seen in the main pulmonary artery in Figure Q89.1B, this must be a communication between the ascending aorta and the main pulmonary artery. The Doppler pattern in Figure Q89.1C also indicates that there is a communication (shunt) between a high-pressure artery (the aorta) and a low-pressure artery (the pulmonary artery). This is not a rupture of the descending aorta into the left pulmonary artery because the flow would be in the opposite direction, as in patent ductus arteriosus. Atrial septum defects would have low-velocity flow, which reaches its peak in diastole and its nadir in systole. In a VSD without right ventricular hypertension, the diastolic velocity is lower than that which is seen here in Figure Q89.1C.

This patient had a large ascending aortic aneurysm (AA), as is seen in Figure A89.2.

90 Cold Leg

This 67-year-old woman presented at another hospital with a cold leg. Workup revealed occlusion of the right femoral artery, and the patient underwent an embolectomy with restoration of flow to the leg. She was transferred to our hospital for further evaluation, on warfarin with an international normalized ratio (INR) of 2.8. On admission she was in normal sinus rhythm (NSR) with a normal blood pressure and respirations. There were no signs or symptoms of congestive heart failure (CHF). A transthoracic echocardiogram was performed (Figures Q90.1A through Q90.1D).

QUESTION 90.1. Based on these echocardiograms, what would you do now?

1. Do a transesophageal echocardiogram (TEE)
2. Increase the warfarin dose to achieve an INR of 3.5
3. Do a Holter monitor, looking for paroxysmal atrial fibrillation
4. Balloon mitral valvuloplasty
5. Mitral valve replacement

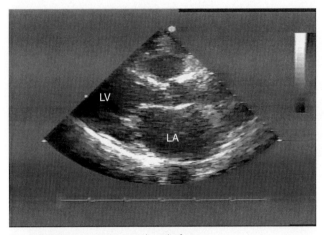

Figure Q90.1A: Long-axis view, diastolic frame.

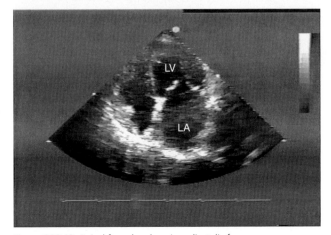

Figure Q90.1B: Apical four-chamber view, diastolic frame.

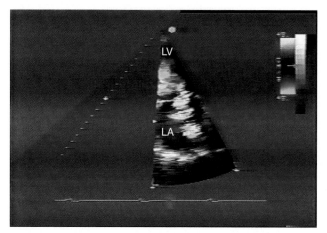

Figure Q90.1C: Same view as Figure Q90.1B, with color Doppler.

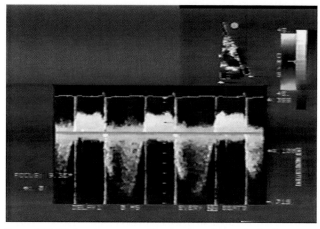

Figure Q90.1D: Continuous wave Doppler through the mitral valve.

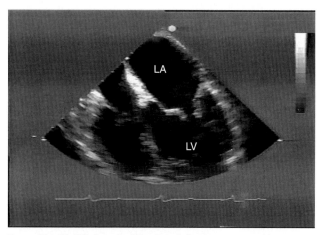

Figure Q90.2A: TEE, four-chamber view, 0 degrees.

QUESTION 90.2. Based on Figures 90.2A through 90.2C, what is your recommendation now?

1. Mitral valve replacement
2. No further treatment is necessary because the patient has no signs or symptoms of CHF
3. Finish the TEE
4. Obliteration of the left atrial appendage with a coil

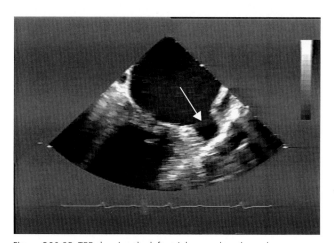

Figure Q90.2B: TEE showing the left atrial appendage (arrow).

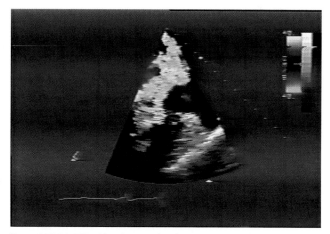

Figure Q90.2C: TEE with color Doppler, showing severe mitral regurgitation.

QUESTION 90.3. There was no evidence of patent foramen ovale or valvular vegetations (Figure Q90.3).

What would you do now?

1. Aortic endarterectomy alone
2. Aortic endarterectomy prior to cannulating the aorta for mitral valve replacement
3. Mitral valve replacement without aortic endarterectomy, and add antiplatelet therapy
4. Something else

QUESTION 90.4. Based on Figure Q90.4, what would you do now?

1. Aortic arch endarterectomy alone
2. Aortic arch and descending aorta endarterectomy
3. Combined arch and descending endarterectomy with mitral valve replacement
4. Make a phone call

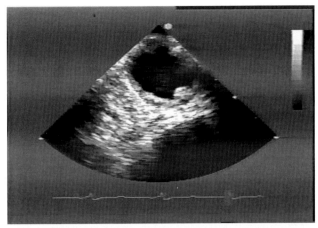
Figure Q90.3: TEE of the descending thoracic aorta.

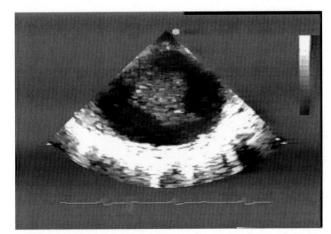
Figure Q90.4: TEE of the distal aortic arch.

ANSWER 90.1. Correct answer: 1, do à TEE. This is an echocardiography book, and therefore doing a TEE is almost always the right answer. It is clear that this patient has mitral stenosis and regurgitation, and had an embolic event. Because the patient is in NSR and has significant mitral regurgitation, the likelihood of a left atrial clot is lower. TEE will offer details about the differential diagnosis. It has not been shown that a higher INR (greater than 3.0) will be beneficial in a patient with mitral stenosis and NSR. Since the patient is already anticoagulated, a Holter monitor will be interesting, but not vital. Balloon mitral valvuloplasty is contraindicated because of the significant mitral regurgitation. Mitral valve replacement may be indicated, but further evaluation should be done first.

ANSWER 90.2. Correct answer: 3. Because this is an echocardiography book, finishing the TEE is the only correct answer! In a more serious vein, one should finish what one starts. Mitral valve replacement is not indicated in a patient with one embolic event, NSR, and no other symptoms. The reason for the embolic event has still not been established definitively because the left atrium and its appendage contain no thrombus (there was also no "smoke").

ANSWER 90.3. Correct answer: 4, something else. The "something else" is to finish the TEE (which we have already established is always the correct answer!). The arch of the aorta also has to be investigated.

ANSWER 90.4. Correct answer: 4, make a phone call (to the other hospital's pathology laboratory to find out what the pathology findings were from the initial femoral embolectomy). The mass in the distal aortic arch is heterogeneous, large, and may not be a thrombus. In fact, the pathology from the femoral embolectomy revealed malignant cells diagnosed as angiosarcoma. Although the patient underwent surgery for removal of the aortic sarcoma, she died of multiple organ failure (embolic in nature) postoperatively.

TAKE-HOME LESSON:
A comprehensive test is a must, even when the diagnosis seems obvious.

CASE

91 Maladie de Roger?

A 45-year-old man, who runs marathons, has a history of a ventricular septal defect (VSD). He was admitted to the hospital with fever for 1 week. On physical examination his blood pressure was 110/70. He had a loud holosystolic murmur at the left sternal border. On transthoracic echo (TTE), the cardiac chambers and wall motion were normal, and color Doppler shows the VSD (Figures Q91.1A through Q91.1E). No vegetations were seen.

A transesophageal echocardiogram (TEE) was then performed to look for vegetations.

Again, there were no vegetations seen, and there was no aortic stenosis or left ventricular outflow obstruction.

QUESTION 91.1. Based on this information, what is the right ventricular systolic pressure?

1. 30 mm Hg or less
2. 31 to 60 mm Hg
3. 61 to 90 mm Hg
4. 91 to 120 mm Hg

QUESTION 91.2. What type of VSD is this?

1. Supracristal
2. Membranous
3. Muscular
4. This is not a VSD

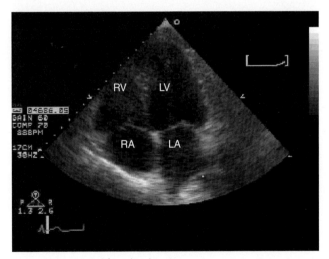

Figure Q91.1A: Apical four-chamber view.

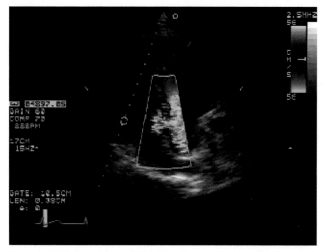

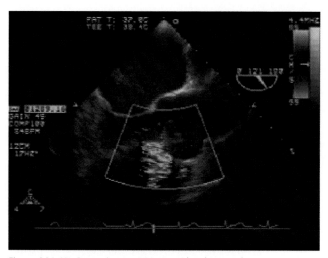

Figure Q91.1B: Same view as Q91.1A, with color Doppler, showing a VSD with a left-to-right shunt.

Figure Q91.1D: Same view as Q91.1C, with color Doppler.

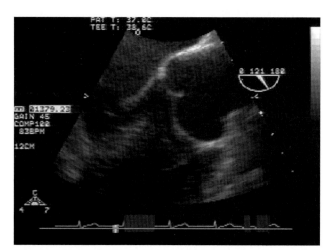

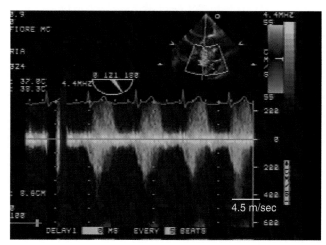

Figure Q91.1C: TEE, 121-degree view.

Figure Q91.1E: Continuous wave Doppler through the VSD jet.

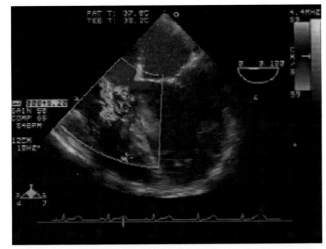

Figure Q91.3A: TEE, four-chamber view, 0 degrees.

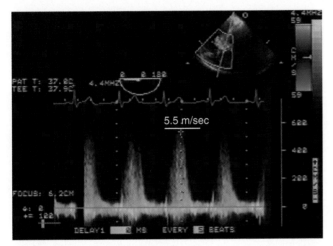

Figure Q91.3B: Continuous wave Doppler.

QUESTION 91.3. During the TEE, tricuspid regurgitation (TR) was noted (Figure Q91.3A). An attempt to measure the velocity of the TR is seen in Figure Q91.3B.

What do you think the right ventricular pressure is now?

1. 30 mm Hg or less
2. 31 to 60 mm Hg
3. 61 to 90 mm Hg
4. 91 to 120 mm Hg
5. I'm confused

QUESTION 91.4. Why is there such a discrepancy?

1. The patient has pulmonic stenosis
2. The patient had septic pulmonary emboli between the time of the TTE and the TEE, and the pulmonary artery (PA) pressure and right ventrical (RV) pressure is really now 90 to 100 mm Hg higher
3. The patient has Eisenmenger physiology
4. The jet that was measured in Figure Q91.3B is not tricuspid regurgitation

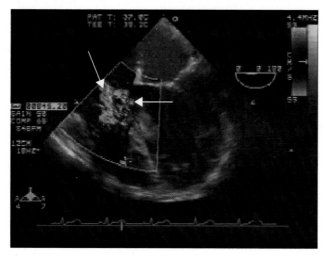

Figure A91.4A: Same view as in Figure Q91.3A.

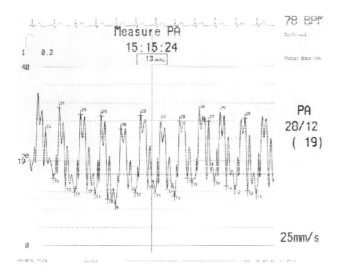

Figure A91.4B: Pulmonary artery pressure.

ANSWER 91.1. Correct answer: 1, 30 mm Hg or less. The systemic blood pressure is 110 mm Hg systolic, and the gradient between the left ventricle (LV) and right ventricle (RV) (calculated from the VSD jet or 4.5 m/second) is 80 mm Hg. Therefore the RV systolic pressure is 110 − 80 = 30 mm Hg. In fact, the continuous wave (CW) jet in Figure 91.4 does not have a completely clean envelope, and the systolic velocity may be even higher (making the RV systolic pressure even lower).

ANSWER 91.2. Correct answer: 2, membranous. This jet is seen just on the ventricular side of the tricuspid valve insertion. A supracristal VSD is located above the crista supraventricularis, below the pulmonic valve. A muscular VSD occurs closer to the apex of the ventricles, in the muscular interventricular septum.

ANSWER 91.3. Correct answer: 5, I'm confused. And so were we. It is hard to explain why the velocity of tricuspid regurgitation now suggests a very high right ventricular systolic pressure: The velocity measured on the CW in FigureQ91.3B is 5.5 m/second, which indicates a gradient of 121 m/second. If this is really the jet velocity of tricuspid regurgitation, the RV–RA gradient would now be 121 mm Hg, and the RV systolic pressure would be 121 + the RA pressure. However from Figure Q91.1E, we calculated the RV pressure to be only 30 (based on the VSD jet velocity).

ANSWER 91.4. Correct answer: 4, the jet that was measured in Figure Q91.3B is not tricuspid regurgitation. If the patient had pulmonic stenosis, the velocity of the VSD jet (between LV and RV) would have been much lower (the RV pressure would have been similar to the LV pressure). Similarly, the patient does not have pulmonary hypertension (from septic emboli, Eisenmenger syndrome, or otherwise) because the gradient across the VSD indicates a normal pulmonary artery pressure.

The jet that was measured on continuous wave Doppler in Figure Q91.3B is not the jet of tricuspid insufficiency. Figure A91.4A shows that there are two jets into the right atrium. There is tricuspid regurgitation (white arrow), but there is also a jet from a shunt between the left ventricle and the right atrium (yellow arrow). The continuous wave Doppler picks up the highest velocity (the lower velocity TR is superimposed). The reason for the high velocity is that the gradient between LV and RA is high.

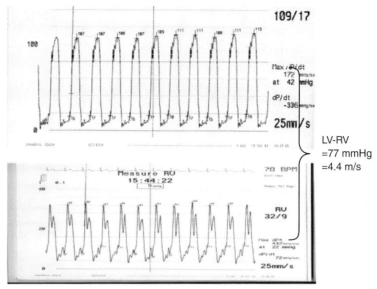

FigureA91.4C: Left ventricular and right ventricular pressures.

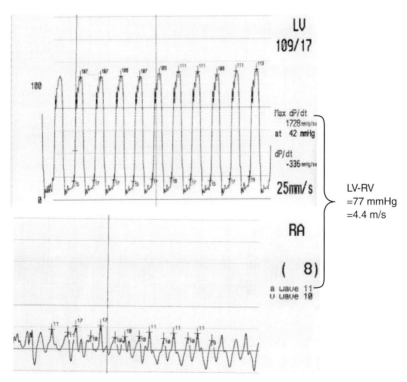

Figure A91.4D: Left ventricular and right atrial pressures.

The patient underwent cardiac catheterization to confirm the echocardiographic Doppler pressures that were obtained. Figure A91.4B shows that the pulmonary pressure was indeed normal.

The right ventricular pressure was also confirmed to be normal, and there was no pulmonic stenosis. The systolic gradient between the LV and RV (across the VSD) was 77 mm Hg, which corresponds to a velocity of 4.4 m/second on the continuous wave Doppler through the VSD (Figure A91.4C).

The gradient between LV and RA (the shunt) was higher, 101 mm Hg (Figure A91.4D), corresponding to the high flow velocity recorded in the RA on the Doppler in Figure Q91.3B.

Finally, oxygen saturations confirmed a step-up in the right atrium (and the interatrial septum was intact). Thus, the final diagnosis is a ventricular septal defect plus a ventriculo-atrial septal defect, and no pulmonary hypertension.

TAKE-HOME LESSON:

People with severe pulmonary hypertension cannot run marathons!

92 Name This Space

A 35-year-old man who is HIV-positive presented with aortic valve endo-carditis and severe aortic regurgitation. The aortic valve was replaced with a tissue prosthesis, and he was discharged from the hospital. Three months later he returned with fever and dyspnea. On physical examination the temperature was 101°F and there was a loud systolic murmur at the left sternal border. A transthoracic echo was obtained (Figure Q92.1).

QUESTION 92.1. What is the diagnosis?

1. Aortic dissection
2. Aortic abscess
3. Ascending aortic graft
4. Right coronary artery arteriovenous fistula

QUESTION 92.2. Note that there is a large amount of flow (aliased, turbulent color signal) into the space in systole in Figure Q92.2A. Figure Q92.2B is a continuous wave Doppler tracing recorded within the space. What do Figures Q92.2A and Q92.2B demonstrate?

1. Flow from the left ventricle into an abscess in systole with severe aortic regurgitation
2. All of the flow that enters the space in systole returns to the left ventricle in diastole
3. The flow that enters the space in systole goes somewhere else
4. There is a communication between the aorta and the space and all of the blood that enters the space in systole returns to the aorta in diastole

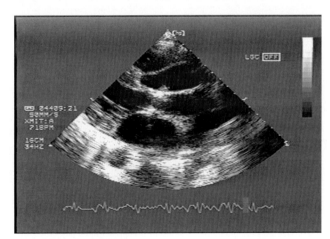

Figure Q92.1: Long-axis view.

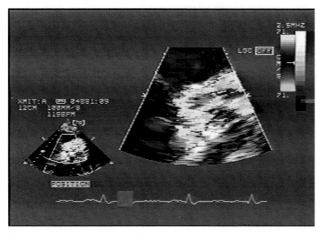

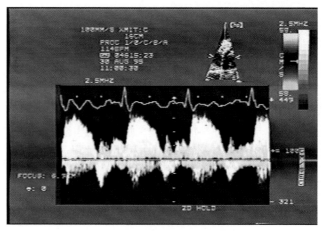

Figure Q92.2A: Same view as Figure A92.1A, with color Doppler, systolic frame.

Figure Q92.2B: Continuous wave Doppler within abscess cavity.

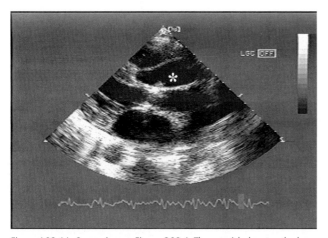

Figure A92.1A: Same view as Figure Q92.1. The asterisk denotes the large para-aortic abscess cavity, which starts at the interventricular septum and extends along the ascending aorta.

ANSWER 92.1. Correct answer: 2, aortic abscess. In view of the history, this patient has an active infection. The history is not consistent with dissection. An ascending aortic graft (which was never inserted in this patient) may give a similar picture, however, the native aortic "wrap," which is sometimes left around the graft, will be attached to the aortic ring and not to the interventricular septum. This is a very large abscess cavity (see asterisk, Figure A92.1A) that extends from the interventricular septum to the ascending aorta.

Note the vegetations within the abscess cavity in Figure A92.1B (arrow).

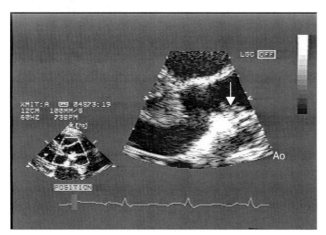

Figure A92.1B: Zoomed view of the long axis.

ANSWER 92.2. Correct answer: 3, the flow that enters the abscess in systole goes somewhere else. Note that there is a large communication between the left ventricle and the abscess cavity (see arrow, Figure A92.2A).

Note the large communication (arrow) between the left ventricle (LV) and the abscess (A).

Also note that the flow signal on the continuous wave Doppler in Figure Q92.2B shows that almost all of the flow in the abscess is in systole (above the baseline) with very little flow leaving the abscess back into the left ventricle in diastole (below the baseline). Therefore the large volume of blood that enters the abscess in systole must leave through another channel. The lack of a large diastolic wave rules out severe aortic regurgitation. It also rules out a large communication between the abscess and the aorta (equal amounts of blood would then go back and forth between the abscess and the aorta).

Figures A92.2B and A92.2C show the communication (asterisk) between the abscess (A) and the right ventricular infundibulum (RV). The flow can be seen to continue into the pulmonary artery (PA). Thus, this patient has a left-to-right shunt (mainly systolic) between the left ventricle and, through the abscess cavity, into the right ventricular infundibulum.

TAKE-HOME LESSON:

Abscesses are aggressive, and may perforate to more than one chamber (fistula formation).

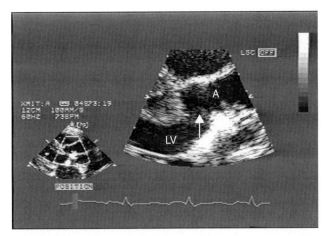

Figure A92.2A: Same view as Figure A92.1A.

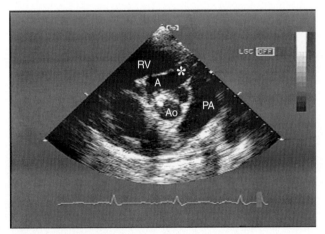

Figure A92.2B: Short axis.

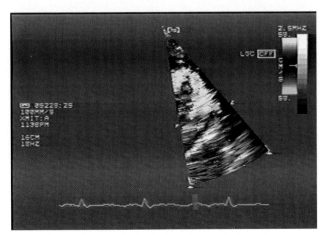

Figure A92.2C: Short axis, with color Doppler, systolic frame.

Index